Faith Christie RN

Jesus. Germs.
& The Great Commission

How I learned to be a nurse and a
Christian at the same time.

ISBN: 978-1-957907-04-8 (Paperback)
ISBN: 978-1-957907-07-9 (Hardcover)
ISBN: 978-1-957907-05-5 (Ebook)

Library of Congress Control Number: 2022943406

Any references to historical events, real people, or real places have been altered and fictionalized to protect the identities of those involved.

Scripture quotations are from The ESV® Bible (The Holy Bible, English Standard Version®), copyright © 2001 by Crossway, a publishing ministry of Good News Publishers. Used by permission. All rights reserved.

Book design by Stephen Porter.

First printing edition 2022. Printed in the United States of America.

Porter Creative
3647 Oviedo
Brownsville TX 78520

www.portercreatives.com

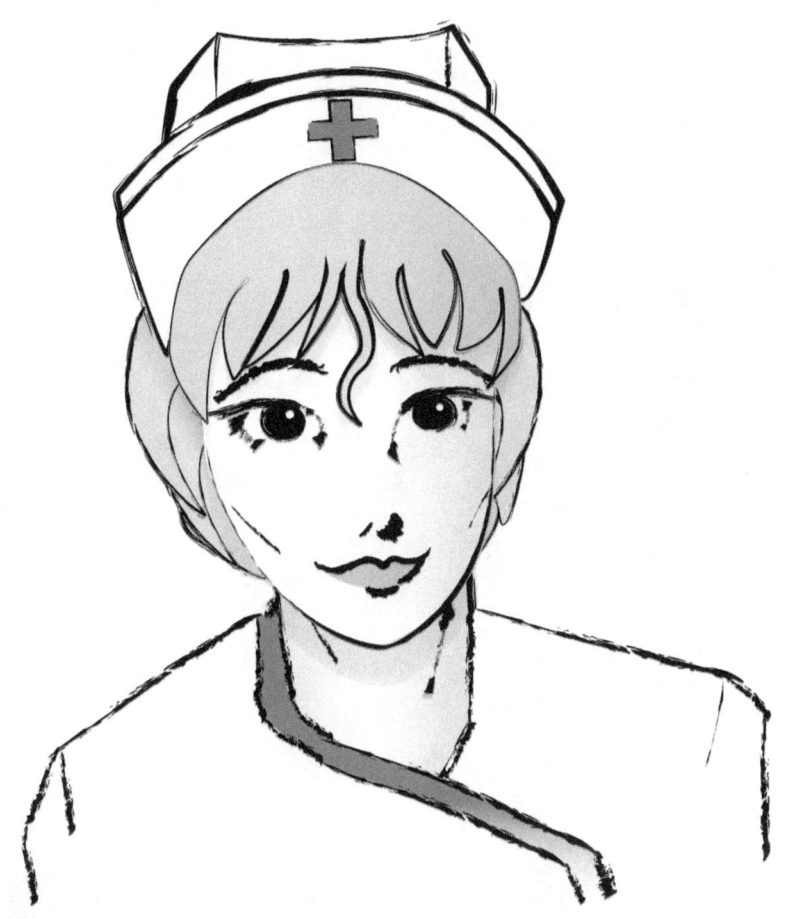

Introduction

INTRODUCTION

Why I wrote this book and how to use it

Although I talked to a lot of nurses before becoming one (and asked enough questions to be irritating), I quickly found out that there was a lot more to nursing than anyone had ever told me. As a new nurse, I searched for a book by an experienced Christian nurse that would help me deal with the spiritual aspects of nursing. I found many faith-based books, articles, and professional journals that told me to keep quiet about my faith because it was "unethical" to share the gospel with the sick. However, there was nothing about how to be a Christian when facing death day after day, the constant lack of closure, or feeling exhausted from keeping other people's secrets.

Now, I understood the fear of acting unethically concerning religious coercion, but the gospel is always unethical by the world's standards, and there has always been opposition to it; Jesus said that this would be the case. In nursing, you could lose your job, but in many nations you could lose much more, even your life. So, the general ethos that I should leave Christ at the door and keep Him out of nursing completely was perplexing coming from sources that claimed to follow Him. And after my search was over, in addition to being incredibly frustrated, I still didn't know how to respond to the real spiritual questions I dealt with everyday as a nurse.

Later, when I searched my memory for the stories that made me feel the most successful as a nurse, or the most inadequate, I found that there was a spiritual thread woven through them. I had learned so much about my faith as a nurse, discovering the humility of Jesus in a whole new way. But I also wished that I had prepared more for my patients' spiritual needs. How could I prepare for what I would face, except by going through it? I wished someone would find a way to tell others how to get ready for this spiritual stuff before they found themselves at the foot of the bed looking into the eyes of a dying woman who wanted to know where her soul would go when she died. What could I do to help?

My answer came when I nearly died during a medical emergency right after nursing school, and the experience taught me how spiritual life and death really are. I realized that I could not begin to respond to that dying woman's request for guidance because I did not understand what she was going through. But surely others could learn these lessons without nearly dying, too? I mean, if everyone had the same spiritual training that I had, the hospitals would be full of sick Christian nurses! How could I help others overcome the deficit of spiritual training in nursing care that was so apparent? I decided to apply the nursing process to my situation to see if I could make a spiritual care plan every Christian nurse could use.

The first task was the assessment: Fear, shame, and an overall lack of experience with death and illness dominated my outlook. I guess that would make the nursing diagnosis some sort of Knowledge Deficit? How about a Knowledge Deficit related to being unfamiliar with sickness and death? The goal of treatment would be to show evidence of a lack of fear, shame, and inexperience, and what better way to gain experience than to go through it? After successfully passing through sickness and a near-death experience, I would totally know how to promote spiritual care for the sick and dying with confidence!

Wait a minute.

We can't just assign a near-death experience to every nursing student—the hospitals would be full! No, there must be a better mode of treatment for this condition. Since my situation was not ideal for large-scale education, and to prevent the educational requirement of mass hospitalization among nurses, I instead assembled a collection of real-life, spiritually-significant healthcare stories and transformed them into parables for nurses and nursing students alike (spiritual case studies, if you will). The patient stories are de-identified for the sake of compliance with the Health

Insurance Portability and Accountability Act (HIPAA): All names, locations, events, and characteristics have been redacted or altered to protect the individuals I encountered, and I have also published this book under a pseudonym to further obscure identifying information. God's role in the events and the spiritual lessons I learned remain unaltered. These spiritual lessons do not require such specific details anyway, and I hope that they can help you learn from my experience without the emotional intensity of the clinical environment. These stories are intended to help you study, reflect, and discuss spiritual care in the nursing role from the safe distance of someone else's life-threatening experiences.

Maybe you're ready to give up like I was. It's okay to admit it. If so, I hope these stories—some beautiful and some painful—will help you sort emotions, understand the spiritual context of this whole nursing thing, and prepare for another day.

It is worth mentioning that my stories do not depict a perfect example. This is not a textbook guide for others to model by any means—I have made many mistakes—but it is an opportunity to reflect on each parable and think about what you would do in the same situation because patients want to talk about this stuff. They will ask spiritual questions as part of healthy development and as part of the natural process of dying, and it is best to be ready for them.

Our patients are an unreached people group in many ways: The gospel is banned, and Christian nurses are punished for talking about their faith or even praying with patients. HIPAA requires that we obscure the truth to protect patients' identities, which is a noble goal, but it also means that testimonies go unshared, and we often fall silent to our patients' sincere questions. That must be why there are so few stories published by Christian nurses—we face the loss of our license and livelihood just for sharing our stories. But we are not alone. There are thousands of Christian nurses working in the field, and often, our forced silence means that they are working right beside us. I cannot count the times I was surprised to find a colleague that I had spent months working with was a fellow believer. Many of us have gone into nursing because of God's call on our life, and we need the encouragement of other believers in this field to remind us why we do it. Even when the details of a story are blurred and erased like in this book, the most important part remains: God cannot be banned from any place, even a hospital, and it is possible to be a Christian and a nurse at the same time.

Today, we are an underground church of Christian nurses, ministering to people who are suddenly aware that they will die someday, and that their eternal souls need critical care. The Covid-19 pandemic has brought this reminder to everyone in the world in a real and powerful way. We pray for our patients, listen to their needs, and help them find the resources they need to push through illness or prepare for the end of their life. Likewise, I pray that God will use this book to help you discuss the spiritual purpose of your work and encourage you in the calling He gave you as both a nurse and a Christian. Discussion questions can be found at the end of each section so that you can ponder what you would do in these situations and seek answers in the Bible. I should caution that some of these stories are like a sucker-punch to the gut and may require some soul-searching, but others are like a breath of fresh air from heaven, reminding us that God is working miracles all around us. So buckle up, and let's get started.

Discussion Questions:

For Individuals or Groups

- What are you hoping to learn from this book?

- Are there any spiritual topics that you try to avoid at work? Why or why not?

Survey Readiness

Special Note

Just like we never know when The Joint Commission will show up to survey our hospital, we cannot know how long we have on this earth. If you do not have a personal relationship with God through Jesus Christ, I invite you to take a moment to pray and ask Him to forgive you and lead your life. The Bible says that everyone has sinned and done what is wrong in God's eyes (Rom. 3:23), and the consequence of our sin is death (Rom. 6:23). But that is not the end of the story: Jesus loves us and died on the cross to pay the consequence of our sins, and He rose from the dead to show that He is greater than sin and death (John 3:16). If you confess that Jesus is Lord and believe in your heart that God raised Him from the dead, you will be saved (Rom. 10:9). For more information, please visit **https://chataboutjesus.com** to chat, text, or talk to someone about becoming a follower of Jesus.[1]

1 Need Him Global (2022). Welcome to chataboutjesus. Chat About Jesus. https://chataboutjesus.com

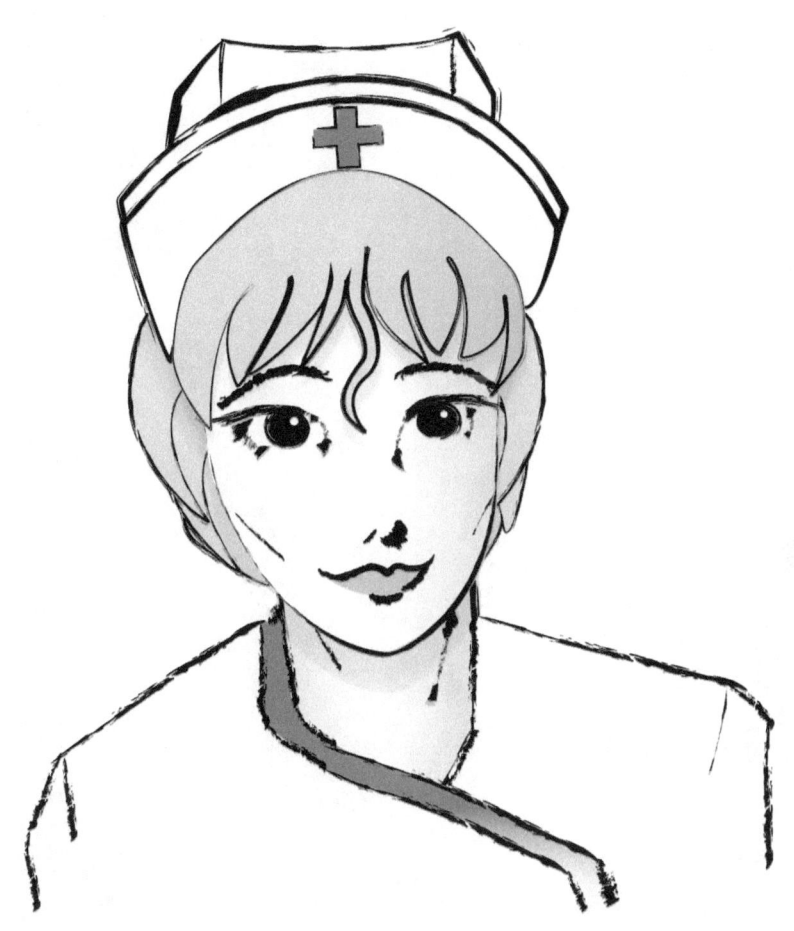

MY STORY

These stories are about my personal journey of overcoming fear to become a nurse

One

Someone Else Should Be Here

I still think about her and her tear-streaked face. She was young, maybe in her fifties, and she was trying to be brave, but it had all broken open; words falling out jumbled, running together with her tears. She was begging for wisdom: "What do I do? The cancer is back—I'm going to die—I just don't know what to do." Then she looked up at me, standing in my student nurse uniform, decades younger and less experienced than her, and she asked me with total trust and vulnerability, "Do you know what I should do? How should I get ready to die?"

I had studied diligently; I got good grades and scored well in my clinicals. But I had no idea how to answer her. So, I just stared awkwardly back at her, my eyes wide as I stepped foot-to-foot in place, wishing I could fade into the wall or run out through the open door. I tried to focus on the picture of yellow flowers on a blue tablecloth above her bed because it felt like I shouldn't be watching her cry, like I was prying into something so personal that I should feel ashamed for looking. My hands felt cold, and goosebumps covered my arms. I hugged myself. People were outside in the hall—people who probably knew how to answer this question.

Someone else should be here, I thought. This woman needs a nurse, a real nurse.

Real nurses could anticipate patient problems like prophets, and I would always ask them, "How did you know that was going to happen?" They always answered me, "I don't know—I can just tell." They had something that I envied: Maybe it was experience? They had seen it a hundred times before. If "X" happens, "Y" always follows. Or maybe it was something about the skin assessment that I was missing? The quality of a breath? A look in a patient's eye? I didn't know. And as my mind wandered through the possibilities of all the early warning signs, so I could stand in the gap against sickness and death for my future patients, a healthy-looking woman was casting the long shadow of death over me and waiting for an answer: How should she face her inevitable end?

I vowed that day that I would either figure out how to work in the valley of the shadow of death, or I would quit and make room for someone better who could do the job.

~

I washed quickly and opened my lunch pack, grateful for a break from the woman who was dying. This was a prestigious oncology unit, but even the breakroom smelled of harsh chemicals, and there were crumbs and catalogues scattered on the worn table. I sat down with a weary sigh and began studying the papers on the walls in the dingy yellow break room. They were covered from table to ceiling with notes, cards, and funeral posters of people who had died on that very unit. Thankful families praised the staff, sharing personal stories of grace and wisdom during their most vulnerable moments, but the eyes of those who had passed stared at me from the posters everywhere I looked. They made me nervous.

In the movie *The Ten Commandments*, Joshua sees death coming to Egypt's firstborn and says, "If it is not forbidden to look upon the breath of pestilence, then see, for it is here."

He holds the door open, but Moses shakes his head and says, "Close the door, Joshua, and let death pass."[1]

The door closes as the angel of death spreads like fog through the city streets. Oncology felt a lot like Egypt that night: Death and weeping were all around, and I wanted to close the door on this clinical assignment as fast as I could, no matter how prestigious it was.

I felt ashamed because I was a Christian, and I should know better. We should run into the fire, not away from it. I should be a shiny, glowy light of peace and kindness or something, right? Instead, I felt like running as fast as I could out of that hospital to breathe real, fresh air. I was too young to contemplate death, and yet I was discovering that as a

---

1 DeMille, Cecile B. (Director). (1956). The Ten Commandments [Film]. Motion Picture Associates.

nurse, I would be surrounded by it.

I swallowed my lunch, hardly chewing, feeling completely overwhelmed. Death and suffering were everywhere. Emaciated bodies, bald heads, and the smell of chemo mixed with sour-vinegar vomit in my nostrils. I had to acknowledge the fear I felt about this place.

The first time a patient died during my shift, I felt so helpless because the look of fear in that man's eyes was terrible; all I had to offer was morphine to comfort him, but it felt like there was not enough morphine in the world to calm his fear of dying. What was he seeing on the other side of those fear-laden eyes? The comfort of a savior, or that other eternity I could not bring myself to think about? Another student shift involved caring for a teenager who complained of severe pain and seemed to be self-destructive. The team of experts found nothing wrong with her, but the family relationship was quite strained, and the patient would smile eerily when her family became anxious about her. It was disturbing to watch, knowing that at some point she could die. I spoke with my preceptor about my concerns that a psychiatric evaluation might be appropriate, and she agreed, but I couldn't shake the feeling that this girl had no idea what she was dealing with, and it could be permanent. Permanent was frightening.

My whole life, I hated making choices; I even ate the same lunch for years just to avoid having to make a choice every day. But I truly despised making choices that were permanent. The risk is tremendous! I was horrified when tattoos became normal because a healthy young person may live decades to see their symbolic image turn into ink porridge. People living in fringe culture can take risks on tattoos because they may not live long to regret it, but now, when we check a new patient's skin on admission, we ask, "is that a scar or a tattoo?" while pulling back folds of blotchy ink to try to determine what the image used to be. But even tattoos are not truly permanent—it is possible to have them removed, though it is difficult. But death lasts forever. There are no takebacks. One mistake, and you lose for good. I finally realized that I was afraid of dying.

I knew the Sunday School answers: Jesus loves you, He died for you; don't die without Him (that one seemed particularly urgent at that moment), but Sunday School answers were not allowed during clinicals. These were the sacred halls of science, and God was forbidden here. I knew that if I talked to the woman about God, I would lose my opportunity to be a nurse, so I racked my brain to come up with the clinical answer to assuage her fears and lead her in the right direction without any scent of coercion. Nothing came to mind.

I prayed intensely that night—for several days, really— about my fear of dying. I confessed it to God and told Him how, as a nurse, people looked to me for answers, how they trusted me to guide them, and I really had no idea what to say. I told Him I was afraid to even talk to people who were facing death, but I knew I needed to talk to them—or at least listen without feeling ashamed and afraid. I asked Him to teach me what I needed to know about death and dying so that I wouldn't be afraid anymore and could be a voice of peace and encouragement to people when they are asking the most important questions. That night, I turned over and went to sleep feeling peace about how I had entrusted my problem to the Lord.

Discussion Questions:

For Individuals or Groups

- What is the biggest fear that you are still holding onto? Why not give it to God now and be free?

- Why do we feel so timid talking about God when someone is dying?

Two

Dying

God does not always answer our prayers the way we imagine He will. I have heard that if someone is afraid of sharks, a well-intentioned loved one might take them on a friendly vacation to experience the beauty of the ocean while they face their fears. They dip their feet gently into the warm water and are encouraged every step of the way until the beauty of the rolling waves and fresh sea air casts away their fear, and they swim with dolphins under the sunset. My experience was not like that. Facing my fear was a bit more like the apostle Peter jumping out of the boat to find a ring of fire over a piranha tank when he expected to walk on water. I cried, doctors uttered expletives, and alarm bells rang out to herald the start of my nursing career. It was an auspicious beginning. Nursing was like God's spiritual shock therapy to deal with the things I feared most.

Soon, I was a new graduate, a newlywed, a brand new nurse, and I was about to be a new mother. I called into work in my last trimester of pregnancy to say that I was "feeling a little rough." I felt like I had the flu and explained that I had a doctor appointment. They gave me a bad time about calling in because our staffing was always "just enough" at the nursing home, and my call-in meant that someone would have to work an extra shift or work short that night. I was in the habit of not confiding how I was feeling because I didn't want to get negative attention from management or something, and they already hated it when a nurse would take parental leave, so I was vague in describing my symptoms. The last thing I wanted was to draw attention to my physical condition, but I felt really ill. I apologized but did not change my mind. There was no way I was going to work that evening.

At my doctor's appointment, the midwife popped in very alarmed. "Do you want to call your husband? He should be here."

My eyes opened wide, "Why? Is everything okay?"

"Oh, well, your blood pressure is very high, your kidneys are not happy, your platelets are low, and your baby has stopped growing. Your baby is actually about the same size he was last month during your checkup."

My heart beat faster. "Is he okay!?"

"He seems to be doing fine, but at 36 weeks and with your blood pressure, we think it would be best to deliver, today. Right away. You should call your husband. Are your bags packed?"

No, of course not; I wasn't due yet, and I felt so tired.

I called my husband and put on the paper gown I was given. That "kind of rough" feeling was getting worse. Somewhere at the back of my skull, a high-school drumline was pounding out rhythmic pain, and I had a migraine-like aura getting bigger by the minute. The room was tilting slightly to the left, so I sat down before I fell, and then I waited for a nurse or the midwife to come and get me. The world had slowed down, and I seemed somewhat distant from it all, as if everything was happening to someone else. Next thing I knew, I was in a new room and hooked to an IV. My husband was there now, holding my hand and saying comforting things, but I could see in his eyes that he was worried. I held his hand back and watched the IV bag as magnesium sulfate dripped slowly into my woozy body. The more drips fell, the more my heart beat erratically. Before long, I was totally woozy and shaky. I felt like throwing up. I thought it was because I had not eaten in hours, but the midwife assured me it was the magnesium.

The delivery was difficult and much of it is still a blur in my memory. I still felt like I had the flu afterwards. The magnesium sulfate infusion continued to make me feel hot, woozy, and shaky, and my blood pressure was still high. I had a headache, but I hoped it was from not having coffee that morning. I said my vision felt funny, but it was probably just the magnesium making me dizzy. Through it all, I kept thinking that when this ordeal was over, I would get to hold my baby and see his perfect little face. When they handed me a squirming blue blob that looked a bit like a wrinkly old man, I could not focus on his features. I smelled his head and held his sweet, warm body close to mine, and I could feel my baby's mouth, nose, chest, fingers, and toes—but all I could see was a fuzzy blue bundle. My head was still pounding, and the room still felt like it was topsy turvy. Everything was dim, and there were a lot of people buzzing around; I had been through a lot that night. I figured as soon as I got home, I would feel better.

But I didn't get better. I got so much worse. When I went to my primary care doctor, they laid me in a quiet room in the dark and told me to rest while they made "arrangements." I felt like they might be preparing my deathbed as they spoke in hushed, worried tones—but I was so tired, I just laid there and closed my eyes, grateful for a quiet rest.

My doctor called ahead and made arrangements at another hospital—a huge research hospital where I was supposed to report to the Emergency Department (ED) and then would be transferred to a bed upstairs. It was the same hospital where I had completed my nursing clinicals. And when I got there, a group of eight residents gathered around me, talking about my case.

"Sh**, she's gonna die."

"Get her out of my ED, she can't die here. She needs a private room upstairs for her village to be with her."

"Yeah, we don't need fifteen people crying in this little room." He gestured toward the curtains surrounding my bed. "Call the house super and get her upstairs stat!"

When I asked the nurse for Tylenol for my headache, she said, "Honey, we have better drugs than that here. Wouldn't you like some morphine?" I said Tylenol would be fine, but again, I could not help but notice a major change in the approach to my care. Was I comfort measures now? Images of Monty Python and the Holy Grail immediately came to mind as I muttered, "Actually, I'm not quite dead yet!"

As it turns out, I had developed a life-threatening complication. My blood pressure was in the 200s, and I was clotting and hemorrhaging simultaneously. The vessels in my eyes had hemorrhaged, destroying tissue, and I was partially blind. I was so weak I could not walk from the bed to the bathroom without stopping to rest. There was a micro-clot in my pinky-finger. I read later that the mortality rate for my diagnosis was 80-100% at that time.

A staff member wheeled me down long chemical-smelling hallways with identical lighting. We rode the elevator several floors, and I remembered what it was like to wait with patients in the elevator, holding my coffee as a nursing student at this very hospital. The doors opened and my bed was wheeled out onto the same unit where I had taken my clinical experience—the one with all the memorials to patients who had died there. Then the transporter confirmed the room with the nurse, who said she would be right in, and wheeled me into a room under a picture of a vase with yellow flowers and a blue tablecloth. He pressed down the brakes on the bed and told me the nurse was on her way. I was now positioned exactly where that first dying woman lay crying, asking what she should do to prepare to die.

My stomach fluttered and my heart rate increased. I was stunned. And who argues with a clean room in a hospital

when it's available? I was certainly not welcome back in the
ED. I had no energy left to care about much, but I did pray
immediately that God would keep me off that papered wall
of memorials in the breakroom. I told the God who made me
that I wanted to live and go back to my husband and watch
my newborn boy grow up. He didn't answer, but I had put my
request on the official record.

Hospitals are terrible at night all alone. I lay in the
hospital bed, and I listened to worship music and prayed for
comfort. My fingers and toes were white from the vigorous air
conditioning at the hospital, and I curled into a ball, trying to
stay warm. My blood pressure increased to dangerously high
levels. A man with a German accent came to my room at two
in the morning to discuss my resistant blood pressure and
how there were signs that my kidneys were shutting down.
In typical Intensivist style, he flipped his long, dark bangs
dramatically, and with a wave of his hand for flare, he ordered
that I transfer to ICU. "We'll accept her now," he concluded.
I wasn't sure if I should feel flattered? While everyone was
busy preparing my transfer, I had this feeling like my body
was fading. My mind and soul were awake and alert, but I felt
like I could step right out of my body. I told my spirit and my
body to stay put, together, and although I felt exhausted, I
forced my eyes to stay open and tried to make conversation
with the staff to keep myself awake. What if I fell asleep and
accidentally died when I didn't mean to?

I silently asked God, "Are we good? If I die now, will you
take me?" I heard—or felt—a quiet, but powerful, whisper:
"Do not fear the one who can kill the body but fear the One

who can kill both body and soul in hell." I knew it was from
the Bible—a paraphrase of Matthew 10:28, as it turns out. In
the passage, Jesus is telling the disciples that they will suffer
for following Him, that no servant is greater than his master,
but that they will overcome it all by remaining in Him.

I chuckled because it wasn't exactly what I would find
on a Hallmark card. I was honestly expecting Psalm 23 or
something pretty and comforting, like cast "all your anxieties
on Him, because he cares for you" (1Pet 5:7 ESV). Instead, I
got "do not fear the one who can kill the body." Man, God can
be a real stoic sometimes! But what I knew in my heart when
I heard that scripture was that if I'm right with God, I have
nothing to fear. I felt distinctly right with Him. Not perfect,
but right. And though He was quiet, I felt He was near and
that I wasn't alone. I knew that He held my life in his hands,
and whatever happened, I would be safe in his care. For the
first time, I was not afraid of dying. I realized that death is not
what I feared most, but only death without Him.

The next day, one of the nurse aides knew me from my
student clinicals, and we chatted like old friends. She washed
my hair like I was a pampered salon guest, massaging my
aching scalp and neck, and brushing my hair carefully into
a neat braid. It was incredible to be too tired for a shower
and to feel so grateful for a clean head. 1 John 4:18 says
"There is no fear in love, but perfect love casts out fear. For
fear has to do with punishment, and whoever fears has not
been perfected in love." I experienced His perfect love in the
hospital—the peace of His Presence and the care of others—
and it changed me.

People had come to my bedside, laid their hands on me, and prayed in the name of Jesus that I would be healed. My prayer chain somehow extended around the world; there were reports of believers in China uttering my name before the Father, and all glory to God, He heard them. A few days later, a dozen expert doctors gathered around my bed and confessed that they had no idea what had happened to me. "You got better too fast," they complained. "We are not even totally sure what was wrong with you."

An older, wiser physician with a gray beard, soft smile and twinkling eyes leaned close and said, "It was a miracle. I'm very happy for you. Go home to your husband and baby."

I knew the source of my miracle!

In an effort to test my ability to discharge, my doctors gave permission to leave the hospital for a few hours to celebrate Thanksgiving dinner, but I didn't live in town. A close friend from church said they planned to be with family out of town for the holiday, so they immediately offered their home to my entire family to host Thanksgiving dinner, and even invited my husband to stay the night with our baby— free of charge. She met with a friend and gathered plenty of chairs and placed the finest tablecloths on the dining room table for my family before leaving to celebrate out of town. We gathered around that God-sent table, eating all of our family favorites, deliciously prepared by my mom and sister, and we gave thanks to God.

Discussion Questions:

For Individuals or Groups

- When has God given you an answer that you did not expect or even want? What was your reaction?

- What are some miracles that you have witnessed in your own life? Take some time to praise God for what He has done.

Three

Blindness

While I experienced a miracle that saved my life, gradually easing into recovery at home, my eyes were permanently damaged, and I had a lot of new struggles to deal with—along with my brand-new infant. I didn't know how I would go back to nursing if I couldn't see clearly to measure insulin, but I asked for prayer from the same family of believers that had prayed me through this far. While the hospital discussed having a Social Worker help me apply for disability benefits on the assumption I would never work again, I thought and prayed about my situation. If God called me to nursing in the first place, then surely He would give me more than a few months to practice; somehow, being a blind nurse would make sense. I finally knew how to be a nurse, and I just knew that an opportunity would come now that I was ready.

It was the middle of winter, and my family had reservations at a hotel near the beach in a faraway state. My husband and I had planned to go along before I got sick, so we timidly asked the doctor if he thought I was strong enough to go on a road trip—with frequent stops—and vacation near the beach with my husband and tiny, new baby. They actually said yes, nodding approvingly at the idea of going someplace warm and being surrounded by supportive family. They said I should take frequent breaks and not get too ambitious, but that it would be fine to go. They gave me their contact information in case of any emergencies and wished us a good vacation.

The first night, I was utterly exhausted from riding in the car for just a couple of hours. I wondered if this was a bad idea. I went to bed at 6pm and slept straight through until morning. I couldn't imagine how sitting in a car could be so exhausting! By the second day, our baby had decided that it made the most sense to sleep during the day in the car rather than at night in the fun hotel, so we struggled with the fatigue of my illness and our infant's needs.

Just the same, that little guy was adorable. He was one month old and filling out beautifully: His wrinkled skin had become plump and peachy. He drooled constantly, stared curiously at shiny objects, and sang joyously about the ceiling fan, giggling all the time. When he slept, sometimes he would startle and whack himself in the face with his own hand. We eventually found a sleeper with Velcro that would tie down his hands while he slept, and it worked like a charm. I could tell by the sound of his cry whether he was scared, hungry, or dirty. I nestled him in my arms much of the day, only releasing him begrudgingly to other family members or for required tummy time. I loved the smell of his head; but I could not see his face. I missed his expressions of curiosity, wonder, fear, and exhaustion. His eyes looked like dark spots on a blurry peach, but I could not look into them the way one looks at someone they love. Sometimes, I missed important details, like a hair wrapped around his fingers, cutting off blood flow to his little fingertips. My husband would ask for my nursing opinion on whether some scratch or rash looked "normal" or "better," and I would scrutinize them with eyes functioning like an out-of-focus microscope and just shrug. I couldn't tell.

Thankfully, the third day of our road trip, just before we arrived at the beach, the sky was sunny and the weather was warm. It felt like heaven. We started early and drove along, sipping coffee all the way, enjoying the warm breeze and sunshine. As we neared our destination, my husband strained forward in his seat trying to catch sight of road signs while navigating traffic in a strange city.

"There—Bella Vista is the next stoplight," I pointed at the street sign.

"Really? I can't read that sign yet..." Suddenly, my husband jerked his head toward me with huge eyes, nearly veering into another vehicle. "You could read that!?"

I glanced back at the street sign, still quite a distance away from our vehicle.

"Oh, my. Yes! I can read it!"

I smiled, still confused. My husband started laughing

and tears filled his eyes as I started reading signs all over the place. Ads for palm trees and alligator shows. Truck parking. Dine-in only. Discount tickets. My husband was bouncing in his seat hollering praises to God while I stared all around at the lush greens and blues around me, taking in the color and detail for the first time in months.

When we stopped, I picked up our son and held him in my lap and just looked at him for a long time, grinning ear-to-ear. The rest of my family arrived, and my husband told them what had happened. They cried and watched me as I watched my son smile and coo back at me. I could see every glorious detail of his God-made gorgeous little face. The next day, my husband spent hours working on a secret project, and soon he called me to the computer to show me something: He had made a video collage of our son's first month, set to his favorite bedtime lullaby. I watched with wonder as his wrinkled old-man-newborn face transformed into the plump baby face I could now see. I found out that he looked funny when he was filling his diaper, and that his favorite toys were a frog from his mobile and a soft flamingo from my friend. I cried because it hurt to know that I had missed those details the first time, and I cried because it was so sweet to know that I would see those details from now on.

I asked God why He made me blind. I complained to Him about not seeing my son's face for so long, and how difficult it was. His answer: "You've never seen My face." I still don't fully understand what that means, except that I am meant to have the same jealousy for God that I had for my newborn baby, and that I probably miss a lot of things that are important to

Him and don't even realize it. Now when I sing the lyrics of John Newton's hymn, Amazing Grace, it is poignant: "I once was blind but now I see." I still cry every time. I know what that's like, and I wonder about what my spiritual eyes don't see yet. It doesn't make me feel superhuman like I thought a miraculous healing might feel—it makes me feel fragile and vulnerable, more aware of my need for God.

When we returned from our trip, I had a follow-up appointment with the Ophthalmologist to talk about my blindness. He conducted a series of tests. He was beaming when he told me, "I have no explanation! This is a total miracle!" God had truly stepped in where medical science failed. The doctor excitedly showed me scans of my eyes before and after, and how my eyes were full of ischemic tissue and hemorrhaged vessels just two months prior, but today they were clear scans. He said, "You can go back to work with no restrictions. You'll have no trouble measuring insulin now."

My healing is just an example of the deposit we have from the Holy Spirit: "In him you also, when you heard the word of truth, the gospel of your salvation, and believed in him, were sealed with the promised Holy Spirit, who is the guarantee of our inheritance until we acquire possession of it, to the praise of his glory" (Eph. 1:13-14). Despite the miracles, I know that one day these eyes will fail once more, and I will face death again. But one day, I will also see Jesus with eyes of flesh when I stand before Him (Job 19:26). After everything I've seen and been through, I can testify that death has lost its sting for those who have been saved by the power of Jesus Christ. The sting of death alone is awful, and if we had no reprieve from it, no hope, the fear of it would destroy our enjoyment of life as well. But I've come to the brink of death, and there is no fear in the perfect salvation of Jesus Christ.

Some people become upset when I tell my story and tell me not to bring my religion to the workplace or to our friendship. I would be lying if I said I did not consider whether the story of God's work in my life belonged elsewhere, but I can't deny that my experience in the hospital bed showed me that there is only one thing that can ease suffering, and that is the forgiveness of sins through Jesus Christ. I am wholly convicted now by this truth, that the Gospel is what is needed most. I am struck by a passage in Acts where Peter and John must answer the Sanhedrin, who have just commanded them not to speak or teach at all in the name of Jesus: "'Whether it is right in the sight of God to listen to you rather than to God, you must judge, for we cannot but speak of what we have seen and heard'" (Acts 4:19b-20). After facing my own death, I never again felt like someone else should take care of my patients; I was finally ready to be the nurse God called me to be.

Discussion Questions:

For Individuals or Groups

- How often do you seek the face of God? He is always there waiting for you and will never turn you away.

- What stops you from sharing your testimony with others? Is Christ not worthy of the reward for what He's done in your life?

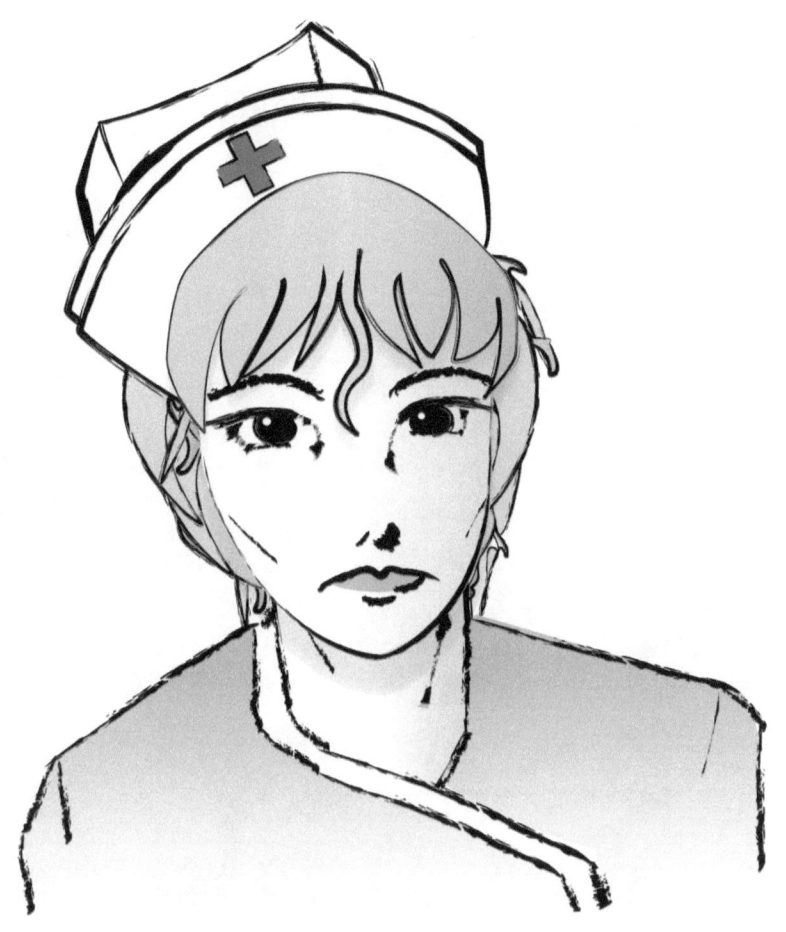

I Should Not Be a Nurse

These stories share how to overcome
weakness as a nurse

One

INADEQUACY

"But the Helper, the Holy Spirit, whom the Father will send in my name, he will teach you all things and bring to your remembrance all that I have said to you." (John 14:26)

I found a seat in the center of an overly air-conditioned auditorium that could seat more than two hundred people. It was packed and the hum of activity carried across the high ceilings. I used to play piano solos in auditoriums this big, but I felt less nervous playing Beethoven than I did right now waiting for class to start. My textbook for this class was so large that I had to slump forward at a 45-degree angle just to carry it in my backpack. I questioned my life choices as I slid back into the seat. With my shoulders crouching forward like a caged animal, I looked side to side, trying to decide whether I should stay and fight or flee like a hunted gazelle.

My sweating palms left water marks across my jeans, and I muttered, "Why am I even here?"

My best friend's words rang in my head, "If you quit on nursing school after all this, I am going to kill you." This statement, and the fact that it was a fiery redhead who said it (I could not quite tell if she meant it when she said things like that) may have been the only consideration that got me into the Anatomy and Physiology classroom that day.

I had been struggling with my calling to the nursing profession for a couple of years already, reading books about heroic nurses and doctors who did such brave things for others—I wanted to be like that, but I had to admit that I wasn't a bit like them. They were good at math and science, they were fit and healthy, they were confident and kind, and they always knew what to do. I took what is affectionately known as "math for poets"—the math class for people who would never have a career that required math again. My health matched my scientific prowess: Any attempt at exercise left me huffing and puffing with asthma after jogging just a short distance with the neighbor's dog. I worried about myself before I thought of others, which often left me paralyzed with irrational worry. I was not "nurse" material.

Yet, there I was, drawn by an invisible and unmistakable force that told me that I was made to be a nurse. I prayed silently as I debated getting up right then and leaving the classroom before the class had a chance to start. "Lord, I have a knack for music and languages, but I am just not good at math and science. I believe I am going to fail this class because I simply don't understand this sort of thing." I suddenly decided it was best to leave and grabbed my backpack off the floor, beginning to stand against its considerable weight.

Just then, the doors burst open, and a distinguished-looking gentleman came into the room, stating in a loud, clear voice, "Most of you will fail this course."

I slouched back down low in my seat, resisting the urge to audibly agree.

Our professor looked like a doctor. He wore casual professional clothes and was crowned with fading white hair and a distinguished beard. He seemed authoritative, and there was an unmistakable twinkle in his eye while he spoke of crushing the dreams of young people. He continued slowly, clearly, and with enough volume to fill the auditorium: "I have made it my life's work to study which students are able to grasp this material and why. I have invested years in perfecting the way this material is taught. In all these years, I have found that two types of people will be more successful than the others."

I waited, wiping my sweating palms, looking down at the floor—just waiting to hear that I did not have enough math or logic or Latin to do well in this class. Memories of my childhood frustration with the multiplication table and long division came flooding back. I felt a bit nauseous, and a headache was forming at the base of my skull. At least now I would have a research-based reason for quitting.

Enjoying the drama, he left us hanging in silence for eons before he cleared his throat and rubbed his hands together. "People who are good at music, and people who have skills in language studies are most likely to be successful in this class. If you play an instrument or find it easy to pick up words in a foreign language, you will have the best grades in anatomy and physiology."

I sat dumbfounded in the chair. The air conditioning began to cool my flushed face, and I shivered.

My professor continued to explain that the kinesthetic skills and spatial awareness of musicians would be helpful in remembering anatomy, and that the Latin words would be more accessible for someone who could take apart the words and "translate" their meaning. Apparently, I was made to be a prodigy in anatomy and physiology. Thank God!

I spent hours reading my textbook that summer. First, I would open the book and find that it looked like nonsense. A sense of panic would wash over me, and I would feel lightheaded. Each time that happened, I would pray that God would grant me understanding because of His calling on my life and help me commit it to memory. Despite my anxieties and poor preparation prior to this course, I ended up pulling a good grade and made some great friends in the process. In fact, my grades were high enough that I had to hide my scores from classmates because they were hunting for the one whose grades "threw off the curve." I found myself really getting into the course material. I actually enjoyed it. I marveled at how mysterious and amazing God has made the human body, and in many ways, my study time became a time to worship my Creator. I started to think, at an intellectual level, that trusting God was going to work out just fine, although I still wondered why He sometimes asked such hard things of people.

Discussion Questions:

- What has God called you to do that you are just not cut out for?

- Was there a time when you tried to obey, and it did not go well? What lessons did you learn from those times?

- If you are living in your God-given calling today, what is more difficult than you imagined it would be? What do you find to be easier than you expected? How has God enabled you in both circumstances?

Two

MOURNING

"**I**f you confess with your mouth that Jesus is Lord and believe in your heart that God raised him from the dead, you will be saved." (Rom. 10:9)

The morning sun shone through my sheer-yellow curtains, warming my room with its light. Living in the frigid North, I was usually excited to jump out of bed and enjoy the warmth of the all-too short summer days before school started. There was only one month before I was starting my new clinical program in nursing, so I felt some impetus to soak up the sunlight while I could, but for some reason my eyes just did not want to open that morning. I would try to drag them up, but they were like garage doors with broken openers—far too heavy to hold up for long. My body felt so heavy. Finally, I let my eyelids have their way and stay closed, but I swung my feet out of bed, determined to go outside with my eyes closed if that is what it took.

My feet touched the floor, and pain shot through them like cold ice; they did not feel like my feet. My eyelids tore open, and I stared down at two puffy orbs at the bottom of my calves. My feet had swollen in the night and were like two medieval maces covered with spikes pointing inward. I took a ginger step and fell backward, unsteady. Clutching desperately at the bed, trying to right myself, I struggled to spread my toes and find my footing. I managed not to go all the way down and stood back up straight. I took a few more steps toward the window. The swelling was subsiding somewhat, so I stood there tentatively moving my feet up and down on the floor while holding onto my bed for support. Soon, I could walk around my room without grimacing.

"That was weird," I thought and turned around to quickly straighten my bedding: that was when I noticed that my hands were stiff and painful as well—my knuckles were swollen, and my fingertips were completely white. In addition, once I was focused on my hands, I realized they were freezing. When I was a child, I used to love playing in the snow, but inevitably, I would lose my gloves and come stumbling home with frozen hands, and that is precisely what my hands felt like at that moment—in the summer. I slid open the curtains and the balcony door and stepped out into the warm, summer sun. It took about ten minutes for my hands to warm up, and I watched with equal parts fascination and agony as blood refilled my fingertips, turning them from white to blue to pink with tingling, throbbing pulses of warmth.

I felt pangs of fear as well. I hoped it was just a weird morning, but later in the day, the same weariness, swelling, pain, and frozen fingertips swept over me in a wave. At a stoplight, I found myself staring at my blue hand, quickly shutting off the air conditioning to make them warm up again. My face and chest were sweating from the heat, but my fingers were blue. It happened again, and again, and each new wave seemed to steal my muscle strength with it. Soon it became difficult to do much of anything. My hands—once strong from playing Rachmaninoff at the piano for hours each day—were too weak to lift a hairbrush above my head to smooth my hair, much less play the piano. Just touching the piano keys sent searing pain through my hands that made it feel like an animal was chewing on my fingertips. My shoulders were so weak and stiff I could not lift my elbow above my chest, and I found that I needed to bend my head down to get my hand up to my head just to make a ponytail with my un-combed hair.

I made an appointment with my doctor. As a young college student, I had only just started going to the doctor on my own without my parents. It was one of those "adulting" skills everyone eventually has to takeover, but most of those visits had been for checkups. Going to the doctor for something serious felt ominous. Luckily, our family doctor was a calm, jovial fellow. He chuckled through his assessments and always had a story to tell. This time when he started listening to my symptoms, there was no trace of mirth in his face. He was worried for me. Terror bucked in my gut like a wild mustang that refused to be ridden. I had read enough in my healthcare prerequisites at this point to know the most probable cause was a crippling autoimmune disease, and images of wheelchairs and feeding tubes flooded my mind.

He shook his head, "At this point, I don't know exactly what's wrong. It could be a lot of things, but it is definitely an immune disorder of some sort. We'll have to do more tests to be sure. I hope it's not vasculitis..." He trailed off, looking away toward his chart. There was gravel in his throat. He swallowed hard and went on to explain Raynaud's syndrome, mixed-connective-tissue diseases, and what I could expect from the labs we would draw that day. Weakness was going to be a way of life from that point forward and would potentially get much worse. There was no cure, but there were some medications that may slow the progression.

I was floored—not by my own weakness, but by the weakness of this profession I had been called into. I had come to believe that medicine was so advanced, disease and death were as rare as unicorn sightings—like something we could flip on and off with a switch. I had never really realized that everyone dies, or that healthcare was always a bit of a gamble. And now my doctor was telling me that the whole medical community was powerless to care for me when I needed them most: The moment I could not take care of myself, all they could offer was to watch and record my decline. And if I could not care for myself, how was I ever going to be a nurse and care for others? Feeling God's call while having my body fall apart before my eyes was terrifying.

The following day, when I could not open an IV bolus wrapper, my nursing instructor cheerily advised me to "Eat my Wheaties" because nurses needed to be strong. My heart hurt, my knuckles throbbed, and I felt so much grief welling up inside, but I just stared grimly at the plastic, thanked her, and walked away to hang the bag. Doubt flooded my brain: With this illness, I wasn't confident I could lift my backpack onto my shoulders, my hands were too weak to grip a drawsheet to lift patients, and I couldn't fathom what my future would be like when I was overwhelmed with just trying to survive.

Meanwhile, I had to ask for help finding the right temperature for bath water because my hands were always cold like the dead. I wished I could have collected a quarter for every time someone would brashly tell me that I'd better start exercising if I wanted to make it as a nurse. This was infernally frustrating since I had grown up jogging, lifting weights, and working hard. I had always thought of myself as a relatively strong woman. I felt that I needed to hide my struggles or risk getting kicked out of the program, so I kept quiet, but I honestly was not sure I could continue. Each day, I wondered if it would be the day my subterfuge was found out, and I would be sent home.

A few weeks later, we were studying autoimmune diseases in class, and there were pictures of someone's hands: They were blue and white. The hands next to them had morphed sideways from Rheumatoid Arthritis. Pain shot through my neck from the sudden tension in my body. I realized I was holding my breath, so I tried to steady my breathing and hold back tears of desperate fear that threatened to swallow me whole. My friend looked over at me from where she was taking notes and touched my arm, whispering with an observatory tone, "your hands look like that." I tried to swallow but my throat was too dry, so I casually lifted my cold water bottle to take a sip, nodding silently: "I know." As I lifted the bottle, someone else commented out loud and pointed at my hands, "Hey, your fingers are blue." I crossed my arms and buried my hands, muttering, "Yeah, it's cold in here. The water's cold." I felt like a hunted animal in that freezing classroom. I wanted to stay in nursing school—felt I had to—but I also felt like the whole world was hunting for the obvious reasons why I didn't belong there.

On one especially bad day, I was driving the one-hour commute to nursing school on a cool autumn morning that was full of sunshine and orange leaves. The rolling hills of fall foliage were so beautiful. I wished I could just stop running so fast, always trying to keep up with a dragging body, and enjoy a nice day. I wanted to quit so bad, I could taste it. I started talking out loud to God, pouring out all my doubt and despair. I could not see how my circumstances would possibly end with me graduating from nursing school. And why graduate anyway? How would I ever care for others if I was sick? What was the point of this calling and all the hard work and pressure? Why was I killing myself to become a nurse anyway?

I called out to God, "I think You're trying to kill me! Why would You tell me to go do this and then hit me with this disease? You know I won't turn against You, but You are going to kill me!" Suddenly, His overwhelming, sees-right-through-and-loves-you presence filled my car. His love for me was overwhelming and palpable. I had to pull over as the tears streamed down my face and blinded my vision. A prayer came from deep within me: "Whatever You are doing, I still want You. I won't serve anyone else. Those other idols can't help me, and I choose You today, even if You kill me. Lead me now, because You are my Master—of everything, forever. I trust You and I'm not going back." I felt like a huge weight was lifted from my soul. I had never said anything like that out loud before. I had never given God complete control over my life, even through sickness and death

Nursing school had several intense exams on how to be comforted by the Lord. That night as I read my Bible before bed, I read the sermon on the mount from the book of Matthew: "Blessed are those who mourn, for they shall be comforted" (Mat. 5:4). I had never noticed that it says "mourn" and not "grieve." Why didn't it say, "Blessed are those who grieve?" I don't mean this disrespectfully, but I honestly wondered if people got points for hurting, or just for volume? I mean, what did Jesus really mean?

After my guttural prayers that day, it dawned on me that grieving is an inward thing—it's frustration, anger, sadness—but all unspoken, the way I hid and harbored all that pain inside myself. But mourning is loud. In many ways, it is a beautiful tribute, like when Jesus weeps at Lazarus's tomb and the people commented, "'See how he loved him!'" (John 11:36b). People in the Bible who mourned would put on sackcloth and ashes and audibly cry out to God, and

He responded to that humility—just like He did when I sputtered my fears and inadequacies by the side of the road that day.

I come from a culture that is quietly productive and very private about emotions. I was totally unfamiliar with mourning. For me, "mourning" became sort of a time of audible confession, and the Comforter came when I asked for help. I started asking for help a lot. I started praying more. It wasn't fancy; it was raw and true.

I would be lying if I said it was easy to proclaim my weakness and needs every day to God. Since that day of confession and commitment, there have been some really tough mornings. There are days that I need to report for work, and I feel like I cannot move because my body is so heavy, and my blood feels thick like molasses. As I drive through the pre-dawn darkness to work with clenched, cold fingers, I sometimes feel more like crawling into a hospital bed and letting another nurse take care of me than walking in with a smile and taking care of someone else. But I pray candidly, now.

Nursing school continued to be grueling and exhausting for me in this awful, weakened condition, but my family, church, friends, and husband all encouraged me, and I graduated from nursing school with high honors, all glory to God. I grudgingly must admit that it all worked out without "my strength." As my pride and self-sufficiency died, His glory made me more like what I was created to be. When I have nothing to give, only His love remains; that is perfection.

Discussion Questions:

- Do you mourn or grieve? Take some time to confess your ugliest needs out loud and ask God for help.

- Was there a time when you surrendered to God totally and completely, even if it wrecked you? Why or why not?

- What is keeping you from surrendering to God totally and completely? And are you ready to give it to Him?

Three

GOD'S FAMILY

"**F**or you did not receive the spirit of slavery to fall back into fear, but you have received the Spirit of adoption as sons, by whom we cry, 'Abba! Father!'" (Rom. 8:15)

My parents were visiting us from out of town, but our vacation time was cut short when I took my mother to urgent care for a medication adjustment. Suddenly, the color drained from her face, her responses became more and more dulled, and she passed out right there in the clinic. She was having a reaction to the medication and was transferred to my hospital, where I was familiar with the doctors and staff. I had floated in this ED from the ICU when the need arose. I knew where the supplies were and all the protocols. I knew the assessments and even what the doctors would prescribe for my mother. I knew she would be admitted—I had seen this same scenario play out countless times, and I was itching to skip the formalities and get my mother the treatment she needed.

Her ED nurse was a tall man with glasses named Aaron, and he was taking excellent care of her. I watched him carefully, ready to speak up if I saw any lapse in best practices, just so I could do something—I was relieved when I saw that I was not going to catch him making a mistake that day; he was flawless in his care. I knew Aaron's work; he had a reputation at the hospital for being one of those nurses that always went the extra mile for his patients. I could tell by the way he cared for my mother, looking her in the eye and speaking warmly to her, that he had been called to nursing just like I had.

What amused me was that my mother was not very happy that I found my calling in nursing; I can still remember the day I told her that I thought God might want me to be a nurse. Our galley-sized kitchen was dark and a little cramped. The meal was finished, but the aroma of meat and seasonings still lingered in the small space. My mother was washing pots and pans when I timidly approached to dry the dishes and float the idea that I was considering a nursing career. My "mama bear" is convinced that her cubs are the most extraordinary creatures that have ever crossed the forest, and because of her tireless confidence, she believes in me, encourages me, and supports whatever hair-brained schemes I come up with—but she has never liked medical professionals. I think it might be a personal grudge for all the missed IVs and other healthcare headaches she experienced as a patient.

"Why would anyone become a nurse? You're smart

enough to be a doctor, and frankly, I think you'd do better giving the orders than taking them. Besides, your handwriting looks like a doctor's," she chuckled. "We don't have a doctor in the family, yet."

"Dad's a doctor," I said cheerfully.

"Yes, but not the kind that helps people," she sighed dramatically and winked.

My father is a professor with a doctoral degree not a medical degree. It was an old family joke. As I rubbed the dish towel slowly around the inside of a copper-bottomed pot, I tried again, "I feel called to do practical work—to help people—I want to physically care for the sick."

She shrugged and said, "You always hated being around sick people. Everyone yells at the nurse even though they don't get to make decisions. I just don't think you'd like being a nurse, and I'm not sure you'd be good at it. I still think you'd make a better doctor," she offered hopefully. While she was disappointed when I signed up for classes, she did not stop me from pursuing nursing.

Truthfully, I was pretty sure that she was right about nursing, and I wasn't sure I would be any good at it. When they say that nursing is "holistic," I think it's because the nurse's role description is so vague that they can be blamed for everything that is wrong in the system. If there were problems with wounds, plumbing, clocks that stopped, missing laundry, staffing shortages, delays, sleepy doctors, printers, or even a lack of fly swatters on the unit, the first solution was to yell at the nurses as though they held the entire bureaucratic health-care system—and the gift of life itself—in their reddened, chapped hands. This is not just a feeling or a perception, it's a fact: One time, I requested maintenance on a broken bed three times only to be written up by my manager for not doing enough about the broken bed. Nurses are supposed to take care of the problem or call someone to fix it and make sure it gets done properly. In addition, large portions of our lives are spent working in the middle of the night (which predisposes us to an early death), or away from our families during holidays, weekends, and important celebrations. This labor is lovingly conducted while being exposed to infectious body fluids on a daily basis.

So why would anyone in their right mind sign up for such stress? I knew that she was right about everything, and I pondered the ups and downs of my career while I sat beside her in the ED: me a nurse, my mother an unwilling patient. She looked disappointed again, though not because of me; she was happy to have a nurse in the family these days, and she often called to discuss family medical decisions with me. But my mother loathed the hospital with fury and passion. Today, she was looking particularly upset to have her family reunion usurped by her health. She kept glancing at Aaron, while he fluttered around her doing his assessment. "I'm fine. I think I can go home now."

Aaron continued working, his face calm. He cleared his throat, and spoke to her, "I'm very happy to get the chance to take care of you, Ma'am." He quickly finished checking her neurologic system then asked, "Did you know that your daughter took care of my mother in the ICU?"

My mother's eyebrows shot up. "Really?" she asked, always

excited to hear stories about her children. She tilted her head at Aaron. I looked straight at him, a bit suspiciously, hoping that it was a good story with no complaints. I steeled my emotions (in case it was a bad report) and squinted at Aaron, trying to remember. Vague memories of the occasion were swimming around in my brain—a large, kind family with lots of unanswered questions and an intubated, distinguished mother—but I could not remember details about her illness or whether she survived. I had taken care of a lot of patients over the years.

Aaron smiled and waved away my confusion. "It was a long time ago—long before I was a nurse even." Turning to my mother, he explained, "I watched your daughter bandage my mother's wounds and clean her, all while tracking those computers around her; I was shocked that a person could keep track of all that stuff and still explain everything to us with kindness and compassion. Your daughter is a great nurse! I told my family at the time, 'I could never do that'—but then I knew I had to. When my mother died the following week, I decided to apply to nursing school. Somehow, I just knew that God was calling me to care for others like that." He turned to me again, "And now I get to take care of your mother, just like you took care of mine. It's really an honor."

Humbled, I looked down at my mother's face and saw genuine pride that what I did had made a difference in this man's life. He was now paying it forward with excellence as he cared for her. No one had looked at me and said, "she would be a really good nurse." What Aaron saw in me that day was not my skills or my training or some inherent talent—it was

Jesus showing through me. Jesus had genuine compassion and love for a family in need of God's comforting Presence, and He had loved them through me.

When Aaron left to report to the physician, my mother reached for my hand and smiled at me with tears in her eyes: "You're a very good nurse. And a good daughter. I'm very proud of you. It's so good that you were there for his family like that."

I squeezed her hand, "and it's a good thing he's here for my family. I guess that's why God called us to be nurses."

My mother nodded with understanding, "to take care of His family."

Discussion Questions:

For Individuals or Groups

- How can a person discern God's will apart from our personal desires?

- What is an example of a time when God used circumstances to affirm His calling in your life?

Four

WEAKNESS

"For it is God who works in you, both to will and to work for his good pleasure." (Phil. 2:13)

Decades later, this cursed disease still plagued me; my fingers were a cold mess, nearly as blue as my royal blue scrubs but with little painful ulcers that screamed in agony whenever I touched anything. I watched myself cry in the mirror, telling that weak woman looking back at me, "Buck up, and forget the pain." She sobbed in reply, uttering desperate words. One of the ulcers had gotten snagged on a sock while I was getting ready for work, and I was doing my best to keep my footing while waves of pain washed over me. Most days, the medicine my doctor prescribed years ago kept me going, and I felt almost normal. My fingers would heal and function like they were supposed to, although it took longer than normal.

But sometimes my immune system would flare, and it felt like a flashback to that summer day when it all went wrong overnight. I wanted to call in sick to the hospital, but I knew that if I started down that road, I would never go back, and nursing is my calling: my sacred duty. Still, it was beyond me in that moment to walk into a patient's room, smile, and tend to their very real needs. I did not have the strength. If I had to go to the hospital, I should be the one crawling into a bed and letting someone else take care of me. I prayed candidly, clenching my jaw at the pain, "God, I can't do it. I simply cannot be a good nurse today, I'm just too weak. I need You to show up, walk in that room, and be a nurse to these patients. They are expecting someone to take care of them today, but I have nothing to give. Either that, or I need to quit. I can't do this much longer."

I was praying with my hands lifted. They were blue and white in color with ulcers flecked across my fingertips. I suddenly remembered an image from a church conference for refugees from Sudan: An elderly woman hunched over a cane with gnarled, crippled hands and scars running up her arms. She stood at the front of the church, and as the worship music swelled, she looked straight up toward heaven with a beautiful smile and raised her crippled hands in praise. She was bursting with joy, scars and all. At the time, I found myself whispering, "I think that's beautiful." I felt a wordless agreement in my spirit, as though God was agreeing, "Me, too." Seeing someone come through trials and worship God was really moving. So I gave my hands to God again, and asked Him to work through me.

I trudged onto the unit with my coffee cup in hand and took report. My first patient was an elderly woman who could only speak Spanish. I did what I could for her and communicated in broken Spanish through pain and fatigue. About midway through my shift, her daughter approached the nurses' station where I was working on charts.

"¿Discúlpame? (Excuse me?)," she said. Like her mother, she also spoke only Spanish.

"¿Sí?" I responded, looking around for backup from another nurse with better Spanish and more physical strength than I had available at that moment. I really did not want to go and do anything for her mother. Exhaustion and pain were crippling me: physically and spiritually. I had nothing left to give, and I was in no mood to hear criticism or needless patient requests.

The woman beckoned me wordlessly to the patient's room. I expected some pillow needed to be moved or some hangnail needed immediate attention, and I walked back grudgingly. When we entered, she smiled broadly and motioned to her mother, who smiled back for the first time that day. The daughter launched into a torrent of praise about how well I had taken care of her mother, who nodded at me in agreement. They would not stop.

I only understood half of what she was saying, but it was pretty clear that she thought I was doing an amazing job as she reached for my aching hands and squeezed them gratefully. I shrank back horrified and ashamed. I shook my head and responded in broken Spanish, "Gracias a Dios por todos. No soy una buena enfermera, excepto con Dios."

(Praise God for everything. I'm not a good nurse, except with God.) How could I take credit for anything good that day? The daughter's smile grew even bigger, and her eyes filled with tears. The old woman raised her frail hands to heaven and spoke out loud, "Gracias, Señor, por enviarme una ángel en mi necesidad. (Thank you, God for sending an angel in my time of need.) I nodded sheepishly, still somewhat confused, and began to nod and praise God with her as the woman's daughter joined in. We must have been quite the sight, praising God in our different languages: a real picture of heaven. The rest of the day, I enjoyed my work. My body still hurt, but it didn't seem so overwhelming because I had deep joy now. I guess I really needed that little worship session to pick me up and help me through the day, and while God worked through me to serve this precious little family, He also worked through that family to heal my soul.

That was not the last day that I felt weakness and pain going into work, but it was the last day I believed my condition would prevent me from being a good nurse. I learned to treat my despair with praise. I continued to pray that God would care for His patients through my weak and sometimes useless body. The same thing would happen, like a song on repeat: Every time I gave up and asked God to take charge, some patient or family member would call me their angel, and they would praise God in heaven that He had sent me in their hour of need—and every time it would bring tears to my eyes, and I would praise God right along with them because He was with me in my hour of need, too. It does not matter if I am weak, or if the medicine I thought was so foolproof turns out to be weak; truly, His strength is made perfect in all my weaknesses (2Cor. 12:9). As my pride and self-sufficiency dies, His glory rises and makes me more like what I was created to be, and I was created to be a nurse who is strong spiritually, not physically. When I have nothing to give, only His love remains: "Not by might, nor by power, but by my Spirit, says the LORD of hosts" (Zech. 4:6). I've come to realize that dependence is my best hour, both as a nurse and as a Christian.

Discussion Questions:

For Individuals or Groups

- Do you hide your weakness? Has God ever seemed to fail you when you were weak? If so, discuss and pray.

- Have you ever tried to put your trust in your own strength instead of God's strength? How did it go?

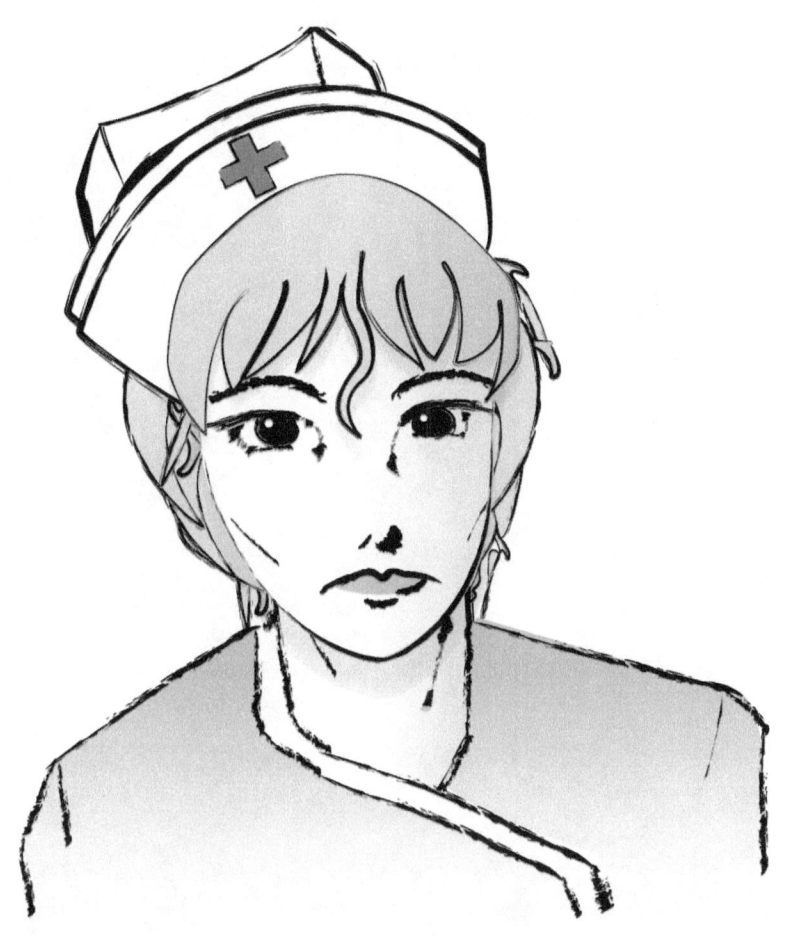

MY FIRST PATIENTS

These stories are about patients who
taught me how to be a nurse

One

THE PRIEST

"Truly, truly, I say to you, a servant is not greater than his master, nor is a messenger greater than the one who sent him. If you know these things, blessed are you if you do them.'" (John 13:16-17)

I was a brand-new nursing student, nervously taking one of my first patient assignments of the year. I was still trying to figure out how to keep a good, organized "brain" with my patient's most critical info from the Kardex and trying to figure out whether highlighters were helpful or just an extra, time-consuming task. The air was crisp and cold with the smell of brewing coffee mixed with disinfectant. My interest was piqued when I found out that one of my patients was a priest in stable condition, and my first job was to help this patient get a complete bath, brush his teeth, and get comfortably up to the recliner.

While the morning hygiene routine may seem like a simple task, there is a "right way" to do everything in the nursing profession—a more clean and tidy version of what you might do at home. For example, there is a correct way to fold the washcloth over your hand—folded in half and wrapped in thirds over your hand for a good, padded grip. There is a right way to test the water temperature with your elbow and pre-warm the soaps in the warm water before applying them to the patient's skin to prevent discomfort or hypothermia. I was instructed on the proper order of cleaning the body, starting with the cleanest places, and moving carefully to the more soiled areas in a head-to-toe fashion. I was taught how to vigorously massage the back to increase circulation and help prevent pressure ulcers. I found out that there are steps to correctly fold the linens, make a bed, line a chair with the drawsheet, and drape towels on a bedbound patient for privacy and warmth. Every detail of a simple bath had a "right way" that was based on centuries of experience. I could just imagine Florence Nightingale flourishing linens with the skill and art of a top chef plating fine cuisine.

I was not Florence Nightingale. I was nervous and clumsy. My water was too cold, I had difficulty opening the soap, I sloshed the basin on the floor, and I got the fresh gown wet within the first two minutes. It was a raging failure by all measures, but I found myself feeling absolutely content. Even delighted?

Maybe it was because, despite my nerves, I couldn't help but notice that it was a gloriously sunny, crisp, autumn day, and I felt right in my soul just being there. In contrast to the bleak, numbered hallways, my patient's room was banked with windows across an entire wall. We could see a sunrise of trees with orange-brown leaves reflected on the sides of glass skyscrapers. Steam poured from giant chimneys on the roof, and lazy pigeons nestled in their eaves to keep warm. Sunlight streamed into the room like it thought it was in Florida sipping orange juice. It was utterly beautiful.

Despite my initial failure at warming and drying, I eventually had my patient sitting up in a towel-lined chair in a clean, dry gown, and I quickly got ready to wash his feet, which he had difficulty reaching. I had laid a prodigious number of towels over the shiny, waxed white floors to handle all of my spills and to try to keep my patient's feet from getting too cold in the frigid, dry hospital air. I had also wrapped him in towels to keep his core warm, and he seemed comfortable, though he hardly spoke as he looked contentedly out the window.

I crouched on the cold floor, my sneakers squeaking, hoping I had finally warmed the water and that my knees would not lock in place as I squatted. I prayed that this patient-priest would not mind my inexperience. Without thinking about it further, I started to work.

As I rubbed his heels, the early morning rays of sunshine felt like a spotlight on us, warming everything around us in a halo of gold. I felt like a beam from heaven was shining down on us. The chill melted away, and I felt inexplicably joyful. I looked at the priest's lotion-lathered feet. I had used too much lotion, and they were all slobbery now. I massaged his cold feet to increase his circulation because I really wanted to do everything with excellence, hoping to compensate for my clumsy performance, but I was still not doing it quite right.

Now, I know there wasn't an actual flash of light, but there could have been, because I suddenly heard that still, small Voice speak to me: "You are washing feet. For the first time, you are doing what I did. You are following Me."

I almost stopped what I was doing. Renaissance paintings of Jesus washing his disciple's feet flooded into my mind with words from Bible verses that were stowed away in my dusty brain. I dropped the towel. I felt like I was washing the feet of the High Priest, Jesus. I looked up quickly to make sure those feet still belonged to the same man. As I glanced up, I saw that it was the same priest, but he had his face turned upward toward heaven with a look of complete joy and gratitude, one hand raised as though in worship, like this sunrise foot massage was the best part of his day—not because of me, but because the Presence of Jesus, the foot-washing Master, who was right there with us.

I was floored. I had gone to Bible studies, I loved prayer, I volunteered in the church nursery, and I had done lots of things that taught me about God. But this—this was the first time I had obeyed His command to humble myself and actually do something He did. What on earth took me so long? In the Bible passage about foot washing, Jesus says,

"'Do you understand what I have done for you? You call me Teacher and Lord, and you are right, for so I am. If I then, your Lord and Teacher, have washed your feet, you also ought to wash one another's feet. For I have given you an example, that you also should do just as I have done to you. Truly, truly, I say to you, a servant is not greater than his master, nor is a messenger greater than the one who sent him. If you know these things, blessed are you if you do them.'" (John 13:12b-17)

While squatting down was a bit difficult, getting some warm water and soap was never hard—but despite Jesus's explicit command, I had never washed anyone else's feet. Ever. But when I got down on my knees on the cold floor and scrubbed between someone else's toes, making a giant mess in the process, I was set free from a piece of the pride that weighed heavily on my soul. That sunlit moment is forever etched in my memory, as a reason to do hard, servant-like things, just like Jesus. He likes those dirty, unglamorous places. And while I learned a lot about God in my inductive Bible study classes, I found that I could know God in a real way through spills and wet laundry and service.

The other thing that made me feel joy was the reminder of God's faithfulness. Instead of judging me and leaving me for disobedience and pride, God worked gently, quietly, almost imperceptibly, in a way that made me love Him more, until I found myself on a cold floor with someone else's feet in my hands. "Now that you know these things, you will be blessed if you do them." I would hate to have missed that moment.

Discussion Questions:

For Individuals or Groups

- How would you feel if you had to wash someone else's feet?

- How would you feel if Jesus washed your feet?

Two

THE PARENTS

"And without faith it is impossible to please him, for whoever would draw near to God must believe that he exists and that he rewards those who seek him." (Heb. 11:6)

The nurses gathered around the doors to the room murmuring with awe in their voices. Like shepherds leaning eagerly toward the door of a darkened manger, everyone on the unit wanted to peek at the miracle inside: Just within the room, a middle-aged couple placed pillows around their twenty-four-year-old son's back as he lay sedated in the ICU. The IV pump beeped softly; a slice of sunlight cut through the curtains, marking a path through the otherwise darkened room.

"It's remarkable," the charge nurse whispered, barely audible over the hum of the ventilator. The adult man lying in that bed was supposed to have a life expectancy of age seven, or maybe eleven if he were lucky. He was born with a congenital disease that would quickly kill him. His parents knew that he would die soon, and they knew it from the day of his birth. He had many visits to hospitals over the years, and this visit to the ICU was going to be his last as the doctor informed the family that there was nothing more they could do for him. Their soft tears showed that they had reached an understanding with this fact and come to accept it decades ago.

Those of us in the doorway knew all of this, and his illness and certain death was certainly nothing new to the staff at the hospital—yet, we stood there, watching with rapt attention as though time stood still. As a group of people who worked full-time providing care to others, we were captivated by this diminutive couple: The quiet husband with his soft-spoken, gentle wife attended to their son's needs all day and all night; they had cared for him like this from the day he was born.

"How did he live so long?" one young nurse asked, her eyes wide. It was the question we all wanted to ask.

"His parents' love," another answered. Murmurs went up as the primary nurse began detailing her admission assessment for the small gathering at the doors: His skin after decades of being bedbound was without a single ulcer or bed sore. He was a healthy weight with full cheeks and good color. His teeth were clean and white. His nails were trimmed, and his hair was combed. They had done all of this—all of his care— with excellence for so many years. They had literally laid down their lives in service to his, and he had never, and would never get up, hug them, or utter a single word of acknowledgement. There was no reciprocation of love from their son, except that he continued to draw breath, and that was enough.

We stood as though we were in the presence of angels and whispered admiration of the tired couple before us. We told them how much we admired the care they had given their son and explained that we could do the lifting now. We told them to sit and just watch us so that they could tell us how he liked his pillows; we recognized that they knew what was best for him. They nodded, sitting down with the weight of two decades, and thanked us, wiping tears from their eyes, holding hands while they prayed and said goodbye to their son.

That must be what Mary and Joseph looked like— exhausted, quiet, knowing from the first day that hello is followed with goodbye and that Alpha and Omega lay merged before them. They had no control of the circumstances, but they willingly laid down their lives for God's plan and loved His Son without reserve; their love glorified the One who is most deserving of sacrifice:

> "And they went with haste and found Mary and Joseph, and the baby lying in a manger. And when they saw it, they made known the saying that had been told them concerning this child. And all who heard it wondered at what the shepherds told them. But Mary treasured up all these things, pondering them in her heart. And the shepherds returned, glorifying and praising God for all they had heard and seen, as it had been told them." (Luke 2:16-20)

Discussion Questions:

For Individuals or Groups

- Have you ever cared for someone who reminded you of a Bible character? If so, describe.

- When you think of sacrificial care, who comes to mind? What did they do that was so memorable, and how does it remind you of God's grace?

Three

THIS DISEASE IS A MESS

"**S**eek the LORD and his strength; Seek his presence continually." (Psalm 105:4)

I remember one of the worst things about being a nursing student is that they made us wear white scrub pants. It was so hard to learn how to be clean and tidy while disposing of body fluids and simultaneously worrying about keeping my white pants spotless. Just trudging through the greasy snow (made gray and brown from traffic around the hospital) made the edges of my pants look untidy. There I was, trying to experience everything I could and still keep my white scrubs in a presentable condition.

My preceptor was a smart, confident nurse. She looked at her task list and orders for the day and announced to me, brimming with joy, "Since you're caught up, you can do the dressings on my dermatology patient. He's got full-body dressing changes twice a day. It will take at least an hour... but you'll learn a lot!" She helped me gather the armload of supplies I would need to conduct the dressing change, and I knocked and entered the dark room quietly. I introduced myself to the patient as a nursing student and said it was time for his dressing change. Would he mind if I changed them? He said that was fine, and I premedicated with his pain medication under my preceptor's guidance. Then I piled the supplies at the edge of the bedside table and pulled up a chair for myself as my preceptor walked out.

I used a LOT of saline rinse to remove the dressings from where they had dried into his many open wounds. It took a good twenty minutes just to remove the dressing from one arm. I successfully cleaned the wound, applied the prescribed ointments, and re-dressed his arm. Only two legs, another arm, and his chest and back left to do. I resisted the urge to sigh, inwardly reminding myself to focus on the patient, who certainly disliked the pain of dressing changes more than I disliked a sore back.

We had hardly spoken. I was quite shy, and anytime I spoke, I was afraid someone would realize just how little I knew and refuse to let me help. But as I began to slowly, gently remove the dressings from his leg on the same side, he blurted out, "I'm sorry I'm such a mess." There was a choking sound when he said it, like he was fighting back tears.

I don't know what came over me, but what came next was definitely not coming from the shy, timid nursing student. I felt a tingling sensation down my spine and for the first time in my clinical experience, I knew exactly what to say—God had written the truth on my heart, and it bubbled up at just the right time. I looked him in the eye as my quiet demeanor melted into intensity and confidence; with a fire in my eyes, I spoke slowly and firmly, "You are not a mess. This disease is a mess, and it's awful that you have to go through this."

Now he really did cry. Big sobs shook his whole body. I prayed silently and gave him time to wipe away his tears. After that moment, conversation was easy. I learned about his career and education, how he had recently been promoted to management, but he was concerned about how his illness could affect his new job: The thought that his own body could derail all that he had worked for was wrecking his confidence. I told him I would pray that his employer would understand, and he said thank you; he would really appreciate that. Later, as I dressed his other arm, I told him how I loved my clinicals but had so much to learn that it sometimes seemed overwhelming. He told me I was one of the best nurses on the unit, and I would be fine. Soon we were both smiling and laughing. I didn't bring that into the room with me—God met us there; both of us were feeling inadequate and needing His reassurance, and we both found what we needed over painful wounds and a mess of gauze. I was a different person when I left that patient's room. God had changed me.

People often comment on how hospitals are de-humanizing, but I have found that illness is the really de-humanizing element: Whether you are in a hospital, a mansion, or laying sick by the side of the road, the part that hurts is the part that was broken since the beginning—the part that makes you not the best version of what you were created to be. Sin and the curse creeps up on us like stains on a white uniform—their presence mangles our fragile bodies, and it hurts like the first time Adam and Eve walked out of that ancient garden of perfection; it is a gut-wrenching loss. The glory of God's image broken, impossible to repair on our own.

But it is not impossible for the One who made us, knows us, and cares for us.

When I met my patients, when I delivered care or watched over their procedures, I started to think of Jesus's body during the crucifixion. He knows about suffering, and He cares. I started looking for Him. Before, I had seen nursing as a chance to be the hands and feet of Jesus, and I still believe that's true. But meeting Him unexpectedly in a man covered with painful wounds awakened the realization that He was there ministering to me, too. Serving Jesus fills me up with His Spirit of joy, peace, and patience, and I would go home from my clinicals with the fruit of the Holy Spirit just spilling over.

Meeting Jesus in my neighbor is a big deal to me because my compassion gets tired sometimes: There are times when I realize how greedy, proud, and ungrateful human beings can be, and it doesn't make me want to break my back to serve them. But when I look in their eyes and see Jesus in the image of God they bear, it doesn't matter so much what the external person is saying or doing. I want to care for His image, whether broken or whole.

Discussion Questions:

For Individuals or Groups

- What tasks do you dread the most?

- What patients do you least want to care for?

- When do you have the best conversations with your patients?

Four

LAUGHTER

"The LORD your God is in your midst,
A mighty one who will save;
He will rejoice over you with gladness;
He will quiet you by his love,
He will exult over you with loud singing."

(Zeph. 3:17)

"Is Clint back from Rehab?" I asked, noticing a familiar patient we had recently discharged from the ICU.

"Oh yeah, and he's as cheerful as ever. He hasn't stopped complaining since he got here," answered the weary night-shift nurse.

I remembered Clint very well because he had the gift of sarcasm. He reminded me a lot of the men I love most: my husband, father, and grandfather, so I understood him and his sarcastic humor. His wife would often say, "Oh, Clint, this nurse gets you! She's gonna dish it right back at you!"

But Clint was having a bad day. He said his stomach hurt. I assessed him and noticed that he was very distended and complaining of severe pain. He tended not to complain about the pain and would just get grumpy and sarcastic, but I knew that his subtle complaints were probably worse than he was letting on. I called the doctor right away, and we talked. Initially, he ordered a stool softener twice a day, but I explained Clint's discomfort and distention and requested an enema.

Wait, what?

You have to understand that any nurse who has done one enema is hoping that it was their last. When the nurse who coached me through my first actual, live-patient enema told me to put on a facemask with a shield, I didn't truly understand. My eyes widened as I saw that she was serious. So, you understand that the level of empathy at work in my normally selfish heart was already quite high when I requested an order for an enema—not to be given on the next shift but administered by moi. It had to be divine intervention. Clint needed some serious relief.

The physician must have realized this was an unusual situation at that point because he said, "Sure, you can do that. And if it gets worse, get a CT of the abdomen without contrast and call me."

I updated Clint on the plan of care, and he sounded not-too-thrilled but desperate enough to comply. "Anything... I'll do anything to relieve this pressure!" he said, gripping his pillow and spinning in the bed again. I resisted the urge to tell Clint that my mannequin had lost a leg during a simple Foley insertion in nursing skills lab. It just wasn't the time.

Instead, I donned my gown, facemask with eye-shield, double-gloves, piles and piles of linen and Chux pads, an enema kit with warm water, and a shovel. (Just kidding about the shovel.)

Clint had surprisingly little to say as I laid the linens down and positioned him. Only once did he ask, "Is this really gonna work, or are you just torturing me for kicks and giggles?" I told him I really thought it would work, but that he shouldn't judge me if I laughed at his farting noises.

I opened the clip and as the warm water poured into his colon, the most glorious thing happened: Gurgling billows of flatus burst out of his poor, pressurized peritoneum. At first, he apologized politely. Then he whispered prayers of gratitude. Then loud, boisterous praises of sweet relief filled the room. "It worked! It's like magic! It worked! How did you know?!"

We sang a happy song, and I danced a happy dance over the bedpan. We made so much noise, you would have thought that a new baby had been born. People came to check on us but left quickly when they saw our face-splitting smiles and the odorous procedure that was underway. It was so strange, this mixture of bodily fluids, horrendous stench, and exuberant joy. We rejoiced together in his relief and gratitude. The best thing about that enema, though, is that I earned Clint's trust. For weeks after that, I was able to talk to Clint like he was a friend. He shared his concerns about how his wife would handle it if he didn't get better. I told him she was soft as silk on the outside and tough as iron on the inside. He laughed, "That's true! You know what? That is true. If she can handle being married to me, then death is going to be a walk in the park to her." He smiled and glanced at her picture proudly.

I believe God wants to talk to us and that He has a wonderful sense of humor. There are times when I take long walks, praying the whole time and chuckling over silly things. Yes, sometimes prayer is just plain fun. When I'm old and gray and someone hears me talking to myself, I want them to say "Oh, she's just praying—she always does that."

A few weeks later, I was working on the unit when Clint passed away. I stayed with his wife and remembered our laughter together after she said goodbye. She told me, "Clint really liked you. He said you were one of his favorites here. I think he knew that you just got him; he could be himself with you. I can be myself with you, too, because I know you really cared about him." She held my hand tightly, telling me that she wasn't going to take time off from work, because keeping busy would help her grieve in a healthy manner. Soft as silk and tough as iron, I admired her, too.

The thing is, I really was going to miss him. The laughter and silly, innocent joy that we shared over enemas and sarcasm is one of those fond memories that probably only a nurse would want to hear—but I'm pretty sure God laughed with us and that He thinks those moments are special, too.

Discussion Questions:

For Individuals or Groups

- What do you suppose God sings about when He's singing over you or your loved ones?

- What sort of things do you think God laughs about when things are silly or awkward?

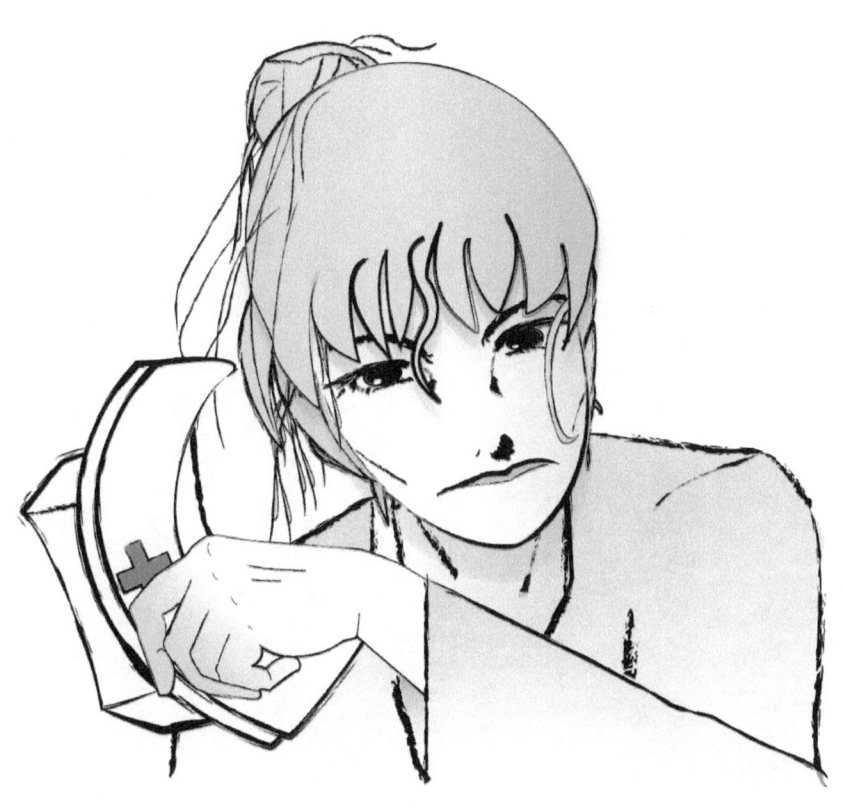

STRANGERS

These stories are about cultural differences, outsiders, and crossing barriers

One

HOSPITALITY

"The second is this: 'You shall love your neighbor as yourself.' There is no other commandment greater than these." (Mark 12:31)

The woman at the checkout counter laughed as a neighboring employee called out something in Spanish. I worried that they were laughing at me. I was thirteen and self-conscious already. Then I heard a derogatory term for my skin color, and the woman at the checkout counter looked down, suddenly self-conscious. I was the only white girl in the entire store. Living in another culture was giving me a case of paranoia. I was going through enormous culture shock; black pepper was considered a "spicy" ingredient where I grew up. I fretted over the color of my skin, hair, and eyes because they were like badges indicating that I did not know things that everyone else understood. Sometimes I grew frustrated with being repeatedly corrected because I was dressed wrong or didn't know about a tradition.

The kindest people, who wanted so much for me to fit in, would put shellfish and hot sauce on my taco, saying "No, that's not the way we do it; this is how it's done." They were trying to be helpful and fix it "right," but I was allergic to shellfish and my tongue broke out from hot sauce. There is no room for objections when you are the outsider, and while I appreciated their kindness, I missed being myself.

At some point, I decided that I could learn to understand the culture and speak the language, but that it was still best if I could be myself within that culture. I did learn a great phrase, however: "Tilt your head, not the taco." If you tilt the taco, all the filling pours out; if you tilt your head, you'll get a nice neck-stretch and an intact taco. Likewise, sometimes I just needed to bend a bit and be flexible with my surroundings and schedule—if not, I would be likely to make a mess. But honestly, I just wanted to go home where things were normal.

When I finally returned to my homeland, I really tried to be friendly to outsiders because I knew how it felt to be different. Once, when I tried to be welcoming, my efforts were perceived as a mockery: One entire group of foreign students told me they thought I was laughing at them because I was always smiling—it was unnatural to them. Even in my desire to help others and empathize with them, I had a great deal to learn! We did become friends, but it took a long time to build trust.

When I started nursing school, we all had bright futures: We dreamt of competitive offers, sign-on bonuses, and paid internships. As I imagined the offers flooding in, I prayed that God would only allow one hospital job offer to come through, so that I would know where He wanted me to go. A month before graduation, our entire graduating class was in tears as we assembled in our classroom. A recession had hit, and all our job offers dried up overnight: No one wanted to train a new nurse without experience. Sure, there were nurse shortages, but hospitals were willing to work short rather than spend money on training during a recession.

"Well, You didn't have to cause a recession to answer my prayer, Lord," I laughed sardonically on the way home. Joking aside, I was nervous. I found part-time work at a nursing home, but I knew that I needed to get hospital experience, or a lot of options would close. After the birth of my son and my recovery from blindness, a new passion to use my skills to the fullest flooded my soul. I started applying to a new job every day. I applied to about fifty different entry-level jobs across the nation and only got three phone calls, which resulted in two job offers in the same city. Guess where? The same Spanish-speaking cultural area I had gratefully left as an awkward teen.

My mother used to tell me not to ever tell God that I would "do anything but," because as soon as I said that I would not do something, He would ask for it. She said, "I never wanted to go to Africa with all its man-eating animals and rare diseases, but I never told God I wouldn't go, because I was sure He would send me if I did!" The single job offer I prayed for was a choice between two hospitals in the same city, both where I had sworn I would never go again. My husband and I prayed and made a choice between the two; we drove to a place where our nearest relatives were 1,700 miles away and where we did not have a single friend. If something went wrong, we were totally alone. I sat on the sofa and cried that first day. How would we make any friends?

We moved into our apartment on Friday and went to a new church on Sunday. A couple at the church were quite friendly, and we hit it off right away—they even invited us to come over for dinner that same week. When we got home, I cried again—this time, with tears of joy. I told my husband, "Honey, we're gonna make it! God has already provided friends." That blessed church couple was so kind to us when we were outsiders. We were just three strangers sitting down to a lovely dinner with believers who followed Abraham's example of hospitality.

And God was wise to send me there: This time was so different because I was no longer a gangly teenager, but a nurse with a desire to work on the mission field, armed with a better knowledge of how to handle culture shock. I wanted to work as a missionary nurse, but my student loans would keep me from going into missions. On this assignment on the other hand, I was able to work and pay off my loans while speaking a foreign language and practicing cross-cultural skills. It was ideal. And the people were wonderful. I remember one of my patients would roll out in his wheelchair to my computer desk with a broad smile on his face to teach me Spanish vocabulary in the middle of the night. He couldn't sleep, and I learned numbers to one thousand, days of the week, seasons, and many other practical words. He celebrated with me when I was able to announce his blood sugar in Spanish and hollered to other patients that I was getting good at Spanish, so they better clean up their language.

Overcoming cultural differences got easier as I studied diligently and showed people that I was willing and eager to learn. I think it helped to be secure in my own identity this time, rather than trying to figure out a new, grown-up identity in an unfamiliar culture; I could invest my energy in learning the culture and language without trying to figure myself out at the same time. My patients also appreciated that I spent time talking to them and listening to stories about their families and traditions, and I started to enjoy this whole cross-cultural experience as well as my new home.

The book of Hebrews says simply, "Do not neglect to show hospitality to strangers, for thereby some have entertained angels unawares" (Heb. 13:2). I can't begin to explain what this verse really means; in many ways, it baffles me—but I know that I have experienced that kind of rare hospitality. When I think of Abraham's experience sheltering three strangers who were angels of judgment, I imagine Abraham must have been really glad he invited those guys for dinner!

Abraham was extravagant in his hospitality, killing the fatted calf and hosting a spontaneous mini banquet for his guests. Some of the most amazing Christians I have ever met were extravagant in hospitality. They rolled out the red carpet, cooked homemade meals after a full day of work, left a basket of snacks and beverages by my bed when I showed up unannounced and in desperate need of a place to sleep, and showed me their "church lady bin" in the back of the car with on-call supplies to make coffee and serve cookies at a moment's notice. I want to be like Abraham and be extravagant like these saints, but in the meantime, I'm grateful that I got to meet some real Abrahams who showed generous kindness to strangers.

In the process of trying to show hospitality (and often failing), I learned who I really am inside—but even better than that, I learned more about God. Kindness is worth the risk because it pounces emphatically on original sin and directs our gaze away from ourselves. My son told me once that there is a character in a Star Wars series who understood his enemies by studying their art. Creation and the people who live in it are one of God's masterpieces. Now, when I reach out to strangers, it is partly because I want to know God more, but I also get these little glimpses of His vast creativity every time I see something or someone different in this wide-open world; it's a new view of the Creator I love. Even an introvert like me can enjoy meeting new people as a representation of the Creator's art.

Discussion Questions:

For Individuals or Groups

- What is a time when you were grateful for hospitality from strangers?

- Have you experienced culture shock? Is there a place, people group, or job that you vowed to never get involved with?

- What is one way you could show hospitality to strangers?

Two

REFUGEES

"And Jesus said to him, 'Foxes have holes, and birds of the air have nests, but the Son of Man has nowhere to lay his head'" (Mat. 8:20)

I have often thought of Jesus's incarnation as the most tremendous mission trip—from heaven to earth, throne to manger, heavenly glow to blotchy flesh. Talk about culture shock! I once mustered up my courage and signed up to help Sudanese refugees, who were pouring into our frozen city because of conflict in their nation. They had experienced quite a significant journey to get there, and they needed help adjusting to their new home. Ironically, many of the skills they needed were the same things I was trying to learn as a young adult, and I doubted whether I would be any help. The volunteer coordinators at my church confidently replied that they would find a place for me to help; there was no getting out of this with lame excuses. I could see that their passion for the mission would quickly outrun my stamina to remain apathetic.

They gave my number to a Sudanese pastor who was hosting a summer family camp. He said that the husbands and fathers had the most difficulty in western culture, which stripped them of leadership and respect particularly in their work, but also in their marriages as their wives began discussing their new feminist independence from their husbands. They had experienced war, sickness, and refugee camps together, and Biblical counseling was critical to getting through the next stage of the crisis: These families were at risk for alcoholism and divorce. The summer camp would focus on strengthening their faith, their marriages, and their families. The pastor asked if I would be willing to help watch the kids, and since that sounded pretty easy, I said, "yes."

I went and shared a devotional on prayer with them and did my best to keep a large class of elementary-age students safe for the weekend. But I quickly found out that I was the student. These heavenly strangers from Sudan taught me something profound about life and God, pulling the veil back on my materialism to show me what really matters. I saw in them an inexhaustible joy. I saw an old woman with scarred, gnarled hands lift her hands and face to praise God with passion and indefatigable stamina. I saw them worship for hours, all the while knowing that many of them had lost their family members and friends to militias, lions, and Nile crocodiles. I desperately wanted to ask about their joy, but I only had short conversations as I continued to keep my eye on the children.

At about one in the morning, they were still in fellowship, singing and sharing meals, asking me if I would like more to eat, encouraging me as I tried to sing along in Egyptian Arabic. It was delicious food, and after talking to a six-year-old in my class, I found out that their youngest children knew more about cooking than me. "Oh!" she cried. "We need paprika! Go and find me paprika, please!" She was playing in the sand with a stick, but I was still impressed because I didn't even know what paprika tasted like.

A question plagued me through the whole conference. I waited patiently to ask someone, and after a music rehearsal, I got my chance. The youth pastor was younger than me but much wiser, so I asked him, "I have everything I need and more, and I do not have the joy you have. How did you all go through such trials and walk away with so much joy?"

What he explained to me that day shook my world. He said, "the Bible says that God inhabits the praises of His people. When you are really in bad shape, when the enemy is attacking and you have no defense, sing and worship God: He will come down as your praise goes up, and He will fight for you."

I questioned him further, "But wouldn't it be a lie if I don't feel worshipful?"

He paused significantly and asked me, "Is God less worthy of your praise just because of your feelings? No, our praise for God is always true because God is always worthy. Your feelings are the lie."

It was utterly life-changing to stop listening to my feelings and gut instincts and rely on the character of God and His Word in times of trouble. There is a comic that I love drawn by Adam Ford where a mother tells her son to follow his heart, so he asks his heart what it wants, and his heart declares its desire: "Sin!" We often say, "I'm going to go with my gut on this," as if some great wisdom can come from split-second luck. But this message of joy and endurance was not dependent on feelings or situations (or even the lack of war), and it has produced lifelong joy in my life. I am so grateful for these "angels in disguise" who came such a long way from home and were willing to teach me the connection between obedience and joy. Just like Jesus.

Discussion Questions:

For Individuals or Groups

- What is it like to worship God when you don't feel like it? Is it ever appropriate to withhold worship?

- What are some worship songs or hymns that are always true about God?

Three

ALIENS

"You shall treat the stranger who sojourns with you as the native among you, and you shall love him as yourself, for you were strangers in the land of Egypt: I am the LORD your God." (Lev. 19:34)

My report that morning started with a political debate about immigration. When I finally got to hear about my patient, I heard that Maria was very young (much younger than me) and had been found by the authorities after getting injured. She was nine-months pregnant, was not a legal citizen, and was already in labor when they found her. She was rushed to the hospital and had an emergency c-section. I was informed that her Hepatitis C test was positive, but that she may not know that yet, and that she may have a post-op ileus (bowels that stopped moving after anesthesia). She only spoke Spanish and, while I had cared for many undocumented patients on the unit, there was some stigma over this patient. I prayed about it and determined that I needed to treat my patient like a cherished daughter of God; I realized that the situation did not change my ethics, and to "do no harm" and "love thy neighbor" was still the top priority. Besides, I had enough to worry about just trying to talk to her about her bowel situation without fluency in Spanish—we would have a lot of extra steps just figuring out the basics of communication and determining when to pull in professional translation services.

I walked in the room to find a young woman, looking left and right with wide brown eyes set in a tense face. She was terrified and looked as though wild animals were chasing her. She was so scared, but she calmed down just as quickly when she saw me smiling. She took a deep breath, and slowly and painstakingly, we used hand motions and my broken, toddler-like Spanish to figure out what she needed at a basic level (water, no ice; lights on; how to use the call-light). I also needed to explain what was keeping her in the ICU. How do you say "post-op ileus" in Spanish? I knew the doctor was coming early, but I wanted to see if she felt the urge to go to the bathroom yet.

"Necessita poo-poo" (you need to poo-poo) I questioned her.

She looked at me with a confused smile.

"Numero dos en el baño" (number 2 in the toilet) I held up two fingers. "Es muy importante. Usted está aquí en el ICU para su estomago. Puede numero dos, puede mira al bébé. Entiendo?" (It's very important. You are in the ICU for your stomach. You can number 2, you can see the baby. I understand?)

I thought she may have understood? Did I have time to call-in to the translator service?

Just then, the surgeon entered. Surgeons, as a group, walk very fast and say very little. A nurse must be ready to record all of the few words spoken, or there will be consequences. This one was downright friendly as he declared, "Take her to see her baby. Grab the monitors, all of it, and take her to her baby. That's an order. When she sees him, she'll go to the bathroom. It's the hormones, you know. The baby makes everything move."

I nodded, thinking that was some funny Labor and Delivery voodoo. But just the same, it would certainly do her some good to see her baby. The trouble is that I had another patient to care for, Maria had several pounds of equipment to take with her, no one was available to help, and the baby's unit was across the hospital, over the River Kwai, and deep into Timbuktu. I had a long conversation about logistics with the charge nurse that morning, and we both agreed on a plan. The charge nurse was going to watch my other patient while I arranged a traveling tower with Maria's monitor and jimmied the IV pole into a pocket of the tower so that I could push both at once without jeopardizing anyone's safety. Then I could push her in the wheelchair very slowly with my one remaining hand, and we would travel across miles of sterile floor and through countless security doors together with our monitor-tower camel.

At this point, Maria and I had become best buddies. We were laughing and sharing jokes on the way to the nursery. I had called ahead, and the nursery staff had prepared a visiting/nursing room for my patient and all of our various equipment where she could privately meet her baby. Everything was going according to plan.

We entered the room and settled in as the nurse brought in a healthy-looking, chubby bundle with tufts of dark hair peeking out. She had huge brown/black eyes that tried very hard to focus in the direction of her Mama. She immediately started suckling toward her mother, and the nurse provided a ready-made bottle for Maria to offer her.

Suddenly, Maria looked up at me, wide-eyed. "Ahora! Numero dos! Aiee!" (Now! Number two! Ack!)

The nursery nurse quickly took the baby as I asked for towels. There was no bathroom nearby for us to rush with that wheelchair; the nearest bathroom was a long, long distance away. Huge bursts of flatus started bursting out, and Mama was worried. I encouraged her and decided I would be happy that her post-op ileus was resolving before my eyes. She was mortified about the whole situation, though, so I started dancing around saying, "Yay! Es bueno! Es muy bueno!" (Yay, it's good! It's very good!) as I prepped a makeshift bedpan with chux pads and towels and helped her sit on a hard chair. She had that confused smile on her face again. She definitely thought I was crazy but seemed to calm down a lot when she saw that I was not angry.

At the end of it all, the "bedpan" was full, the wheelchair was dripping, there were puddles on the floor, and her tummy looked like she had lost about twenty-five pounds. I smiled really big and said, "Se siente mejor? Es muy bien!!" (You feel better? It's very good!)

She smiled too, shyly answering, "Si, gracias enfermera! Discúlpame" (Yes, thank you nurse. Excuse me). I helped Maria first—donning a gown and double-gloves, I cleaned the wheelchair, washed her, and settled her back into the wheelchair with a fresh gown. Then I washed the visitor's chair and wheeled her out to the anteroom while I quickly mopped with towels and cleaned the furniture, floor, and surfaces with disinfectant. I quietly explained to the baby's nurse what had happened as I washed up, and she notified the Environmental Services team that the room needed to be disinfected. Meanwhile, labor and delivery nurses wordlessly began passing perfumed air freshener around the unit to hide the smell.

Later that day, the same surgeon rounded on our unit and said, "Ah, you did well, Miss ICU. I was afraid you were going to ignore my orders but see how well she is now? Everything works better when they can hold the baby. Transfer her to Women's; she no longer needs to be here. You did a good thing today." He patted me on the back and swept out in a flurry.

I felt immense satisfaction. All of that work, all of that effort, and then I had the privilege of taking her back down that long hall to postpartum where she would have access to her baby, without ICU visitation rules to get in the way. When we said goodbye, it was with an awkward and child-like embrace. Despite the language barrier, I believe that neither of us will ever forget the other. It was so hard just to talk to each other, but sometimes the hardest things are also the most satisfying.

Discussion Questions:

For Individuals or Groups

- How can someone show kindness when there is a language barrier?

- Describe a time you were able to cross a barrier and show kindness. How did you feel going into it? What did you learn?

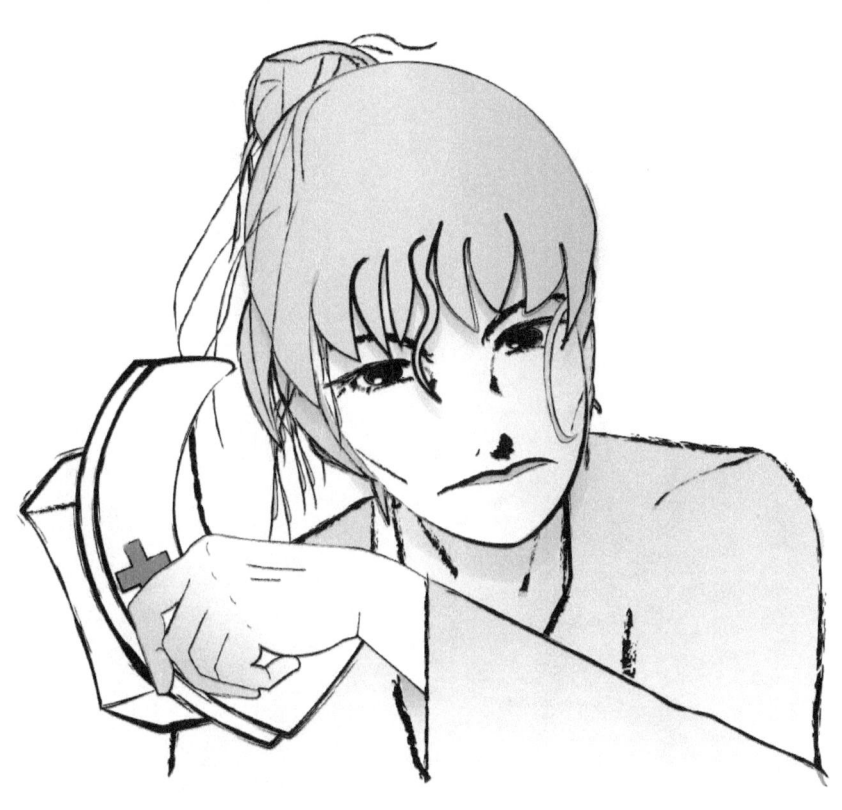

FORGIVENESS

These stories are about forgiving others,
making peace with God, and dealing
with hate

One

PEACEMAKERS

"**B**lessed are the peacemakers, for they shall be called sons of God.'" (Mat. 5:9)

"Judge not, and you will not be judged; condemn not, and you will not be condemned; forgive, and you will be forgiven.'" (Luke 6:37)

When I started out as a scared nursing student, afraid to look my patient in the eye in case their mortality might be contagious, I didn't realize what a precious opportunity it is to be with patients at the end of their life, as they prepare for their death. How often, in any other career, can someone talk about the deepest regrets and greatest joys in their life as they near the end of it? One of the most common concerns for these patients is about broken relationships and the need for reconciliation. As a Christian, reconciliation is something that I'm enthusiastic about.

I used to struggle with forgiveness. A lot. I would pray about it and say, "I forgive you," but I have a stellar memory and am capable of a lot of hurt feelings. I hated being that way, and I did not want to become a bitter person. But I felt like I just hadn't figured out the whole forgiveness thing, and it's a very helpless place to be captive to negative feelings, spiraling toward bitterness and anger. It sounds a lot like that whole sin problem, right? I realized that I needed to ask for help, so the next time I prayed I asked God to help me forgive because I couldn't do it on my own.

Of course, the best example of forgiveness is when Jesus faced His death; the crucifixion is like a cheat sheet for anyone facing bitterness or death. Jesus boldly asked, "'Father, forgive them, for they do not know what they do.'" (Luke 23:34a). When Jesus was attacked, He not only said "I forgive you," but He said "Father, forgive them..." Why would He do that? God promises to judge and punish evil, but Jesus asks Him to forget about it and show mercy.

There's another story like that in the Bible: In the early church, an exceptionally good, really awesome Christian named Stephen models this same request for the Father's forgiveness when he is about to be stoned to death by enemies of the church. The Bible tells us, "And falling to his knees he cried out with a loud voice, 'Lord, do not hold this sin against them'" (Acts 7:60). Stephen not only forgives his enemies, but his last act in this life was to ask God to forgive his enemies as well. Again, why would he ask God to forgive them? Isn't it enough to say, "I forgive you," like we said as children when we hit each other? Am I the only one who felt satisfied in forgiving my enemy because I knew that my heavenly Father would still smite them later?

Out of the blue (and right after I prayed for help), my brother started a conversation with me about the scripture verses above. He explained that we should forgive, but also ask God to forgive others—it was sort of a way to let God know that I didn't want vengeance but would like to see my enemy get saved, just like I was saved. For example, it helps to look at what Jesus and Stephen didn't say: They didn't say, "I forgive them, but I look forward to seeing what You do to them for hurting me!" Instead, they interceded for their enemies so that those sins would not keep their enemies from being saved. This is a crucial detail because a man named Saul (the Apostle Paul) was in the crowd of enemies who stoned Stephen, and God forgave him and called him to preach salvation to entire nations. Forgiveness is powerful stuff! Since Jesus and Stephen both asked God to forget the evil done to them and withhold judgment for that sin, the gospel is proclaimed throughout the earth to everyone who has ever done wrong. We're all in that boat (Rom. 3:23). I sure hope that people I have wronged are praying that God would not hold my actions against me.

And so, I prayed and asked God to forgive the people that hurt me, and it was like a weight lifted off my shoulders. I started praying for their salvation. After insisting that I had forgiven someone (all while struggling to see any difference in my heart), I no longer had to struggle. After that realization, I've come to see this process of helping people reconcile as the real peacemaking work of this temporary life: Reconciliation with God and others is essential if we're going to live in the Kingdom of God without bitterness; heaven is for the forgiving and forgiven, and bringing peace on earth and goodwill to men has a lot to do with interceding for our enemies to get right with God. I think that's why they call it, "making peace with God." Being a peacemaker is about helping others forgive like Jesus does.

Discussion Questions:

For Individuals or Groups

- What do you think it means to be a peacemaker?

- What enemies could you pray for today?

Two

RECONCILED

"**P**recious in the sight of the LORD is the death of his saints." (Psalm 116:15)

I had the privilege of caring for Olivia for several weeks in the ICU. She was dying and cancer had wracked her body. Earlier, she was unable to speak due to the need for mechanical ventilation. We gave fluids, blood products, and vasopressors to maintain her blood pressure. She was bleeding heavily, and it was an uphill battle, but it worked—for a while.

We all felt proud when she was extubated and weaned to minimal vasopressor support. But the cancer was still there, quiet and incurable, and we knew her body would turn for the worse again. That was when I met Olivia's father: Her father was an athletic-looking man who looked years younger than his daughter. He was a pastor and his heart was burdened for the soul of his daughter, who had lived "a rebellious life" of drinking and partying. He told me, "It just doesn't seem right for a father to bury his daughter."

I looked at the woman in the bed and wondered what was in her heart. Father and daughter talked many hours during those days, and as they talked, we had a precious chance to help: Olivia had not talked to her sister in decades. They had a huge fight many years ago, and neither had spoken to the other from that point on. Well, after much discussion, Olivia's father finally convinced her to seek forgiveness from her sister. We flurried into action, happy to do something that would make a difference for her heart and soul when we could do so little for her body.

A colleague dialed the long-distance number, and I held the phone for Olivia to talk without getting short of breath, offering encouragement. This tough-looking woman looked timid and fearful. What if her sister said no? What if this was just going to be another argument? We listened as Olivia gave a heartfelt, humble apology. She confessed that she had treated her sister wrong and was too quick to get angry about little things that "no longer mattered." We couldn't stop the tears in our eyes when her sister told her she loved her and that all was forgiven. Later that day, we called the chaplain as Olivia announced that she was ready to confess her sins to God and get right with Him before it was too late.

There is a beautiful urgency at the bedside of the dying: Father, sister, and God reconciled in the space of a few days. How long do we take to accomplish the same? Everyone will die someday, but when someday becomes a marked day with a deadline, things quickly fall into a category of important, urgent, or not.

One Tuesday, I came to work a little early—something that is unusual for me, as I typically fall through the doors with a giant cup of coffee at the last minute. My co-worker smiled and said, "You're just in time. Olivia is almost there. You can help me sit with her while I call her father." I quickly donned an isolation gown and gloves and entered the quiet room. Olivia's breathing was ragged, and there were staggered periods of apnea. Her swollen body was clean, with fresh sheets and plenty of pillows to elevate her jaundiced limbs and offload pressure. My colleague had done a beautiful job preparing her. I pulled up a chair, lowered the bedrail, and sat with her. I picked up her yellowed hand in both of mine and prayed and watched. I started humming to help her breathe calmly. Her body relaxed, and her breathing became softer. Then I started singing a prayer:

"The weight of pain and sadness gone;
Thank You for forgiveness found.
Close your eyes to the heavy world,
Rise and stand, no longer bound;
Walk into the arms of Jesus."

I looked up just as her heart stopped on the monitor.

One day, if the Lord tarries, I would like to be on the cheering team in heaven, singing a loud welcome song as the saints who live after me come home to eternity with Christ. But on this side of heaven, I think holding the phone to Olivia's ear and cheering her on as she finished well is one of the greatest things I have ever had the privilege of doing.

Discussion Questions:

For Individuals or Groups

- Read Ephesians 4:31-32: What would it look like if you forgave your enemies the way God forgave you?

- Have you ever helped two people reconcile? How did it go?

Three

I'M NOT DEAD YET

"**F**or if while we were enemies we were reconciled to God by the death of his Son, much more, now that we are reconciled, shall we be saved by His life." (Rom. 5:10)

Mr. Livingston had a sour look as I passed by the room. Before I ever took report on him, I could read the bitterness etched on his face. As soon as I walked into the room, he made a sarcastic comment, "Oh good, are you the next nurse that's going to pretend to take care of me by checking her email today?" I ignored his comment and introduced myself, letting him know how he could reach me with the call light after discussing his goals for the day.

In report, the day nurse said that he had informed her of a funeral fund he had set aside so that he would not be a burden to anyone when he died. She was afraid he was expressing suicidal ideation, and I was charged with investigating further. When we spoke, he denied any thoughts of harm to self or others, but he reiterated that he didn't want to be a burden because he knew his ex-wife would not want to "deal with that." I seized the opportunity: "It's good to be financially ready for that possibility. Anytime you are in the ICU, it's a good thing to ask yourself if there is any unfinished business. At some point everyone dies, and whether this is your time or not, it's good to think about it and be ready—without regrets. Is there anything else you want to talk about, to have peace about whatever may happen?"

He shook his head defeatedly, "Well, I feel like a lot of that is out of my hands at this point," he confided. "My ex-wife hates me. My son will have nothing to do with me. At work, I was a tough manager who never cared about anyone—only money. I've really failed in all the important areas. I wish it wasn't this way, but I'm afraid no one will care if I die."

"Well, sir," I said, taking his hand and sitting on the edge of the bed. "It doesn't look like you're dead yet." I paused for effect. "There is still time to apologize for wrongs. There is still time to make new relationships. If you are so blessed to get better and walk out of this hospital, what would you do with your life?"

He answered immediately: "There are all these kids—a lot of dumb young men just like I was—living all around my house. I wish I could have a legacy in this world of being a mentor and making use of all my mistakes. I could warn others to make the right choices and be the father-figure that

I wish I'd had. I really wish I had a chance to invest in the next generation like I failed to do for my son."

"Have you ever tried getting to know those young men around your neighborhood?" I asked innocently.

Mr. Livingston's eyes locked on me. He squeezed my hand. "You've hit on something. I've had it in my mind that my chances were over, but, as you say, I'm not dead yet!" He smiled for the first time. "What was your name again? Well, Faith, I'm going to start living again. I can't change what's done, but I can get busy making things right."

That afternoon, he called his son and his ex-wife and apologized for not loving them the way they deserved. They were cold and did not receive it well, but Mr. Livingston just said, "It was for me more than for them anyway. I've made my peace; I admitted I was wrong." Then he began making plans for a barbecue at his house where he would invite all the neighbors. He told me, "I need to start spending some of my time and resources on the folks around me. We will have a great party!"

I knew when Mr. Livingston discharged because he left notes through physical therapists, physicians, nurse's aides, and anyone else he saw, to tell me that he was going to do what he should have done a long time ago, and to say thank you for reminding him that he's not dead yet.

Discussion Questions:

For Individuals or Groups

- What have you learned from your mistakes? Who else could learn from those mistakes?

- Does your "neighbor" have any problems that you can help with?

Four

SISTERS

"Jesus, knowing that the Father had given all things into his hands, and that he had come from God and was going back to God ... began to wash the disciples' feet and to wipe them with the towel that was wrapped around him." (John 13:3, 5b)

One of the most sickening situations I faced as a nurse involved taking care of two sisters who came in as trauma patients. They were teenagers, and they both liked the same boy. That night, while they were walking down the road, a fight broke out between them. One sister stabbed the other sister, severing a major artery. They were both injured in the fight, and they both needed intensive care, so they were admitted together almost next door to each other.

Their family members were in shock. The girl who was stabbed was struggling to survive and teams worked on her in and out of surgery throughout the next few days, just trying to stabilize her. But the one who committed the assault was there for observation and was doing well overall. She would sit and stare angrily, with utter hatred, toward her sister's room. She seemed to be overcome with hatred, anger, and murderous malice. This was the sister I was assigned to care for all day.

When I could literally see the result of her hatred right across the hallway, it was hard to treat this young woman with compassion. It was so difficult that I stayed in the report room to pray before I went in. When I got report, the charge nurse said it was a tough assignment emotionally and that she could watch my monitors if I wanted to prepare a bit. I agreed, admitting, "Knowing their story, I just need to check myself and pray for a minute, so I do it right."

She nodded and said, "Take your time."

The thief on the cross. Foot washing. The Good Samaritan. All the stories I knew started to flood my memory. God started to remind me what He rescued me from. I knew I needed to offer grace and peace to another sinner, and I didn't want to be angry and unforgiving as if I had never been forgiven. I needed to remember all the sin and darkness that threatened to overcome my own soul before He saved me, so I could carry redemption with me, and maybe, it would overcome all the hate in that room. I remembered that I belonged to God, that I had access to His Spirit, and that I was going back to Him to answer for my thoughts and actions. I was ready.

The young woman so full of hate did not repent or get

saved that day, and she was difficult to care for—very aggressive and profane. She asked how her sister was doing with a sneer on her face, and I confessed that I didn't know. I didn't want to talk about it either way because I felt like she was hoping for the satisfaction of hearing that her sister was dead. I claimed HIPAA and stuck to it.

It was an awful, heart-rending shift, but God helped me be kind to her. Other nurses, techs, and volunteers started asking me, "I read about what she did in the news. How can you be so nice to her?" It gave me a chance to answer simply, "I'm a Christian. God forgave me, now I belong to Him and forgive others." Their eyes widened with surprise as they walked away thoughtfully. Some people remembered what I said and returned to me for advice, prayer, or confession. Knowing that I would not judge a malicious murderer made them feel safe talking to me about spiritual things. I thought I was serving one person, but God was sending a message to others who needed Him just like me.

What if I had been rude to this patient? It still helps to see God's image in others, but sometimes that image is horribly broken. Sometimes it is screaming profanity and full of (literal) open wounds and filth, and sometimes it seems like there is not enough medicine or enough bandages to cover up all that brokenness. When Jesus faced that kind of utter brokenness, just before His own disciples betrayed Him, He did something unexpected:

> "Jesus, knowing that the Father had given all things into his hands, and that he had come from God and was going back to God … began to wash the disciples' feet and to

wipe them with the towel that was wrapped around him."
(John 13:3, 5b)

There are times when we cannot see what God can see, and we must cling to the fact that we belong to God: We are coming from the God who made us, we are going back to God one day in heaven, and the God of the universe can provide everything we need. Nothing else matters. When God looks at brokenness, He knows how to fix it. It's not even a puzzle for Him—it's easy. That knowledge can give us strength to continue serving others when they are ugly and hateful. Half of loving others is seeing His image in them, but the other half is remembering that we are made in His image, too, and that adoption equips us for every task He puts before us.

Discussion Questions:

For Individuals or Groups

- What do you feel ill-equipped to handle when caring for others?

- How does knowing that you belong to God, and you are going back to Him change the way you relate to difficult people?

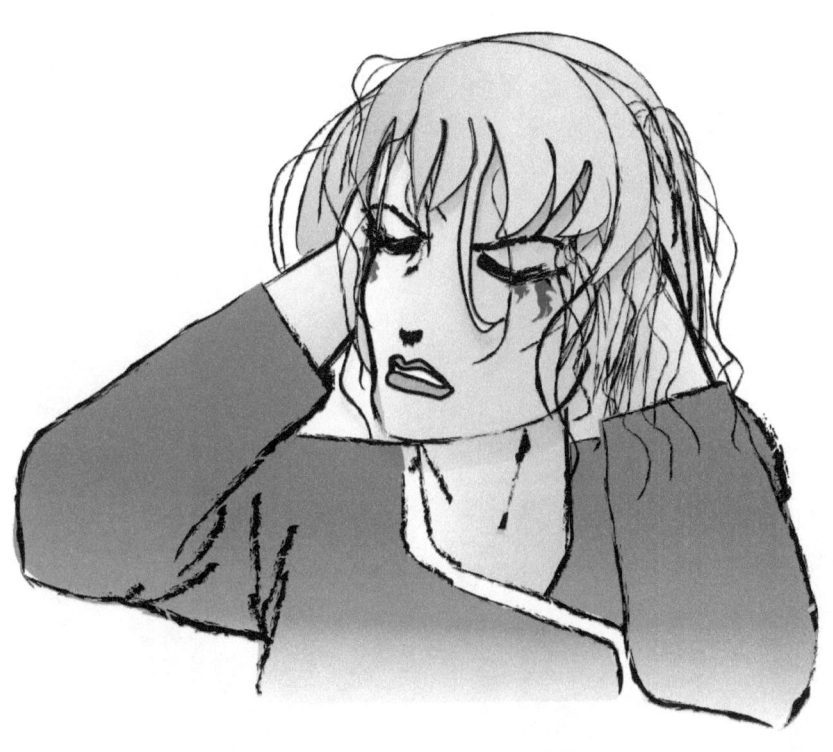

INSPIRATION

Stories of people and moments that inspired me

One

GRANDPA'S BLESSING

"**D**o not cast me off in the time of old age; forsake me not when my strength is spent." (Psalm 71:9)

My grandfather was an eloquent man. After his father was miraculously cured of alcoholism in an old-fashioned tent meeting, the entire family devoted themselves to preaching and holding city-wide tent meetings. Grandpa preached to large crowds of people on a regular basis, telling stories, and explaining the Bible so that anyone could understand. He learned to play the guitar by ear and started playing lively Gospel music to draw people in, then preached until they came to the altar.

The grandchildren of those converts have talked to folks in those rural areas who said their entire towns were saved as the fruit of God's ministry through my grandparents. It's kind of like having Billy Graham for a grandpa—all the kindness and righteousness of a humble servant of God mixed with delightful mischief and laughter. Though a strong man, he would weep when he spoke of how he prayed for us every day, pleading that we would grow up to love the Lord like he did. And other times he would tickle our ribs, rub his rough, five o'clock shadow on our cheeks, play catch, or hide candies and toys for us to find.

In his later years, he suffered multiple strokes. It was awful to see his frustration when one of those strokes affected his speech. He had "word salad" aphasia, and his words came out in a nonsense jumble. "Garden tic-tac," he might say, instead of "Good morning."

"Good morning," I greeted my grandparents. I had come over to their nursing home before lunch with hot coffee to share before heading off to my afternoon college classes. Grandma and I would chat about boys, family, and books, and Grandpa was mostly silent—but he still seemed happy to have company.

Grandpa sat in a wheelchair in a cozy sweater with a fleece blanket in his lap, and my grandma looked small in a giant automated recliner. In the mornings, my grandparents would often sit at the piano and sing hymns to the delight of other nursing home residents—Grandpa sang the melody and Grandma sang the harmony while playing the piano from memory. As they aged, though, it became difficult to come up with the words and chords, and they opted for Gaither videos to start their morning worship session. They watched the same VHS tapes over and over, but they would tell us happily,

"The Gaither's were so good this morning!" Nothing could steal their joy.

When I worked at the nursing home, staff and family members would always leave the TV on in the room. The residents often did not seem to care about having noise in the room, but it seemed to bother their younger caregivers to leave the room so quiet. Consequently, there was a point in the evening when every television in the nursing home was set to a forensic murder series, ghost stories, or seductive shows. I could not fathom that these members of the Greatest Generation would want to watch those shows, but there was nothing else to watch. I realized then that it must have been very refreshing to see my grandparents huddled around Christian comedians and Gospel music, singing along together.

Grandma was always reading a Christian romance book and would slip a folded Kleenex into the book to keep her place. A decade later she developed memory loss and dementia, and she began reading even more. When I asked her what she was reading, she smiled cleverly and said, "I'm re-reading all my favorite books because I don't remember how they end—it's like reading them for the first time! Will they get married, or not? I don't know!" She threw her hands into the air as we dissolved in laughter. She had discovered a secret benefit to memory loss, and I loved her for it.

That chilly autumn day we drank our hot coffee until our tongues were burned raw and we laughed a lot. Then we prayed for each other before I left—they would pray for my classes, and I would pray for their physical therapy or for other family members that they were concerned about. When I reached for Grandpa's hand to say goodbye, my jaw dropped when he took both my hands with great intensity and looked me in the eyes, smiling ear-to-ear, speaking clearly and solemnly from memory:

"The LORD bless you and keep you;

the LORD make his face to shine upon you and be gracious to you;

the LORD lift up his countenance upon you and give you peace." (Num. 6:24-26)

Grandpa could speak! How did he do it when he couldn't say "good morning" without mixing up the words? I locked eyes with my grandmother, whose warm, brown eyes had also filled with tears, and thought how surely God does not forget us when we are old or weak. Both of my grandparents devoted themselves to hours in the Bible, memorizing entire chapters of scripture even in their retirement, and I realized that this was the stuff that lingered when so much was lost: Blessings. God is so faithful. My Grandpa's human strength was subdued by sickness, but I got an incredible glimpse of heavenly strength in that divine moment.

If I could only speak the things I focused on most, what would I be left with? Movie phrases? Memes? Small talk? Or prayers and blessings and truth? I made a promise to myself that I would focus on whatever is good, true, noble and beautiful so that these things would be left with me when everything else fades away (Phil. 4:8). I wanted to be just like my grandparents and keep close to the things that mattered most.

I wiped tears from my eyes, hugged my grandfather
a long time, and thanked him. He patted my hand again
and immediately returned to the jumble of words that
were normal for him at this point. He was the picture of
meekness—humility and restrained strength—the perfect
place to display God's glory. I told him I would never forget
his blessings.

Discussion Questions:

For Individuals or Groups

- What would you do or think about if you could not talk?

- Have you ever been afraid of aging? What would change your opinion?

- What do you talk about most?

Two

STORMS

"'Which of these three, do you think, proved to be a neighbor to the man who fell among robbers?' He said, 'The one who showed him mercy.' And Jesus said to him, 'You go, and do likewise.'" (Luke 10:36-37)

My first shift at the hospital was scheduled to begin just six weeks after we moved to a coastal town and started orientation; a hurricane was schedule to arrive three hours into my shift. My husband and our six-month-old would be sheltering in place without me, and we were distraught to be separated. My supervisor called ahead to discuss the emergency plan with me—I was to bring a sleeping bag, pillow, food, and clothes to last several days until the next shift was able to travel safely after the storm. No family would be allowed to shelter at the facility, but I was reassured that our apartment was in an area with good drainage to prevent flooding.

"Okay," I said, "I've been in floods, tornadoes, and high winds—but what do you do when they happen all at once? Do we go down to seek cover from wind and tornadoes, or up to shelter from floods? I'm just not sure what to do . . ."

My supervisor assured me that my family would "likely" be safe and that the hospital was "pretty sturdy," but I will admit that I was nervous taking my very first solo shift during a hurricane. My co-workers reminisced about a previous hurricane when rats came into the hospital seeking shelter from the floods, but "it wasn't too bad." I was officially terrified. We decided that my husband would drive me into the shift rather than leave the car parked on a flooded parking lot or have him risk being stranded alone with the baby and no vehicle. Rain pounded on our windshield and the roads were already flooding so that cars could only drive down the higher center of the street. The wind bent palm trees sideways as I tried to loosen my tense jaw.

I arrived at the hospital a few minutes early—we left time for detours if needed. My supervisor greeted me, "I tried calling you, but you didn't pick up."

"I'm sorry, the rain and wind were pretty loud, and I guess I didn't hear it ring."

"Well, I have good news for you. The charge nurse on the alternate shift said she would come in for you tonight. Your next shift will be three days away and everything should be clear by then. You are free to go home and stay with your family," she smiled. "I didn't want to promise anything, but I knew you wanted to stay with your baby."

I was stunned by such kindness. Not only was my boss letting me off a scheduled shift, but a stranger was stepping in to cover for me. Then I remembered—my husband had already driven away in the storm. My supervisor quickly rose from her chair, "Oh, I can drive you home. I was going to pick something up at my sister's house, and she is near your apartment."

And so, my new boss drove me home in a hurricane on my scheduled night to work. That is crazy kindness! I can tell you that I had a lot of loyalty toward that supervisor, and it set a precedent of putting others first that helped shape the culture of the unit in a positive way. I wondered if there were others like her?

Years later, a man was transferred to the ICU after a procedure. His wife was exhausted after being up all night, and since they were on vacation, the streets were unfamiliar. When we said he would be asleep all morning and that she could go home to get some rest and a shower, she suddenly began crying and anxiously confessing, "He drove us here with an active heart attack because I have not driven a car in over fifty years!"

My co-worker didn't miss a beat. "I'm getting off in about 15 minutes, and I wouldn't mind giving you a ride home."

"But it's more than 40 miles away! That is certainly not where you are headed already," she objected.

My co-worker insisted, and we handed off report quickly so that she could bring the patient's wife home safely to the hotel where she knew her friends would help her.

Another time, a veteran was found collapsed on his porch from heat stroke and dehydration. When the social worker investigated, they found that his home was uninhabitable and that his only salvageable possessions were the clothes on his back. The social worker arranged for veterans benefits and transfer to a local veterans nursing home, but the best part was when the nurses on the unit played a summer version of secret Santa: They brought shoes, slippers, clothes, an electric razor, and reading glasses for the man while he slept. He would look so curious when he discovered each new gift, studying it curiously, but he never asked, and no one ever told him what was going on.

One of the more urgent stories involved an elderly man who woke up from a stroke with a startled cry: "What day is it? Where am I? My dogs, my dogs!" As it turns out, he had two dogs at home who were likely going without food or care because no one else knew that he was in the hospital. At his age, these two little dogs were his only family, and he was so distressed to think of what they might be going through.

The nurse called the man's apartment manager who agreed to let her into the apartment after receiving verbal permission from the patient himself. We arranged lunch-hour coverage of the nurse's patients so that she could drive to the man's apartment, feed his dogs, clean up after any accidents, and discuss ongoing care of his pets with the apartment manager. The patient, manager, and nurse were able to make a plan where the manager would let a close friend into the patient's apartment twice a day to care for the dogs until he got home.

When she returned, the man was so happy and grateful. Tears filled his eyes when she showed him pictures of the dogs to show their well-being. They talked about his dogs the entire day, and when she left the room she said, "that man is going to get well in no time at all. He is going to get well for those adorable little dogs that are waiting for him to come home." She was right; he did.

Sometimes these inspiring stories involve unusual heroes: One Sunday, a friend shared an alarming story with our Sunday school class: She was driving to her prenatal appointment in Mexico when a shoot-out between the drug cartel and the Mexican military began just around the corner from the side-street she was driving on. She parked the car and hid down by the floorboards of the car, praying that God would spare her life and the life of her un-born son. She made it safely and praised God for protecting her from the infamous cartel.

Some time later, this same woman's husband was driving home from work one night near the border crossing when it started to rain violently, and he lost control of the vehicle, crashing suddenly. He was totally unconscious. His wife sobbed as she described how he was rescued: Members of the same drug cartel drove by him, stopped, and called-in the accident to the authorities. Then they carefully removed him from the vehicle in the pouring rain to protect him from oncoming traffic. When he awakened briefly, they told him help was on the way. They did not stay to greet the police, but the nursing staff said he would have bled to death if they had not reported the accident promptly. Again, they praised God for sending good Samaritans from the criminal underground to save her husband's life.

These are stories that remind me of the inherent dignity of each and every human being. We are made for God, and He has a calling and purpose for each person on the planet. We are not inherently good, but redemption in Christ makes it possible for sinners to glorify a holy God.

Discussion Questions:

For Individuals or Groups

- When was a time that you were surprised by kindness? Have you ever surprised someone else with kindness?

- Would you rather be relieved of something you are dreading, or given a nice gift afterwards? Why?

Three

RAPID RESPONSE FUNDRAISER

"**S**o if there is any encouragement in Christ, any comfort from love, any participation in the Spirit, any affection and sympathy, complete my joy by being of the same mind, having the same love, being in full accord and of one mind. Do nothing from rivalry or conceit, but in humility count others more significant than yourselves. Let each of you look not only to his own interests, but also to the interests of others. Have this mind among yourselves, which is ours in Christ Jesus." (Phil. 2:1-5)

I have to say that when I feel led by God to give generously, I often ask if there will be enough left over for me. I guess it's the sin syndrome of the Prodigal Son's Brother in Luke 15: If we kill that calf for him, will I still have an inheritance? But God's accounting is bigger than my anxious fear. He owns the cattle of a thousand hills, I'm told

(Psalm 50:10), yet when I look down, I can only see what I have in my hands. He feeds thousands with a few pieces, but I worry that if I give away my leftovers, I might get hungry later. The scripture says that if I've ever been comforted by God's love, I should think of others before myself and share that love with them. Especially in the workplace, that can be a tall order.

I was new to the ICU team when I met Joy, but I knew I would never forget her when I heard her next door to me through the drawn curtain, singing over a trauma patient while she skillfully administered blood products and medications. This patient was "bucking the vent" as ICU nurses call it, and alarms were going off constantly as he bit down on his breathing tube and strained against the IV lines wrapped around him like vines. His blood pressure was dangerously low, though, and giving too much sedation too quickly could cause him to crash. As she sang sweetly to him, I heard the alarms gradually calm down, and I knew the patient was improving.

Joy wore colorful scrubs, had boundless energy, and could sway a crowd of people with her wit—either to laughter or to outrage over some injustice. I remember thinking it was really odd one day when I found out that she was missing work. She never missed work. I texted a mutual friend to check on her and found out on my lunch break that she had been in a serious car accident. It was so sudden, and she was in tremendous pain. When I finally got to speak to her, she said she was worried because her contract did not include health insurance benefits.

My own family was short on money at the time after having a new baby discharge from NICU, but I really wanted to do something for her. I thought maybe I could give my time to help—put something together that would be an encouragement to her. So, after work that day I got online and messaged a couple girlfriends from work, asking, "Should we try to do something for Joy? Like signing a card and contributing to her expenses?" I closed my computer then, said a prayer for her, and went to bed.

The next morning, I checked online to see if my friends replied. I discovered that my message had become a group, including nurses, former colleagues, physicians, and friends. While I was sleeping, they decided they could make more money by holding a fundraiser. They also discovered that Joy could use immediate help to cover urgent expenses, so the fundraiser needed to be done in the next 10 days, and I was apparently in charge as Treasurer. The group went viral in our community and nurses from multiple facilities collected donations from their entire work crew at all the major facilities in town. Physicians approached us during our shifts that week to contribute wads of cash: "For Joy—but don't tell anyone it was from me."

When the fundraiser was completed, we wanted to go together to see Joy, but everyone had to work, and they decided I should go ahead and visit her alone to present the fundraiser monies to her on time. I brought pictures from our online page and told her about all the people who were involved, how they loved and missed her, and hoped she would get better quickly. There were hundreds of posts and donations. We raised enough to help with her immediate personal expenses for the month while she could not work. I told Joy that all the money was raised in just ten days and that it was a miracle. I told her we could never do that on our own. I told her that God saw her and loved her, and that He sent all these people at the right moment to help her because He loves her. She allowed me to pray for her, and we cried together, both of us clueless as to how all these blessings came together. She confided that she had felt really depressed being a patient rather than helping others, but that she knew now how much she was loved. I'm happy to say that she recovered fully and went back to work in the ICU again, singing over her patients in her favorite colorful scrubs.

Seeing my co-workers act like family was a big deal to me. In nursing school, we read articles about how "nurses eat their young" and that bullying could be a real issue at work, sort of like hazing. When I started work, I was ready to focus on my patients and not expect anything from the team around me. However, one of my first days in the ICU, I took report on two patients: One was very unstable and needed emergency surgery, and the other was thankfully quite stable on the same dose of pressors all night. Just when the other shift wrapped up report and left, I saw blood on the blanket of my stable patient and found that he had moved his arm and dislodged his IV with the pressors running. As his blood pressure started to drop, I tried to flush his second peripheral IV to switch the drip, but it did not flush. He had no IV access and his blood pressure continued to drop rapidly. The charge nurse paged me to answer the phone and take orders from the surgeon arriving soon for my other patient, and I asked if she could take the orders. She agreed and as tears welled up in my eyes, I brushed them away furiously, so I could see clearly to attempt a fresh IV. I missed. My other patient's ventilator was beeping, and I could tell he needed to be suctioned, as well as prepped for surgery. If his surgery was delayed, he could die.

The charge nurse walked over with a portable phone and gently asked what was wrong. I told her I felt like I had to choose who lives or dies, and I didn't know what to do: Both my patients needed me. She answered calmly, "Oh, don't worry—I'll get this IV started. That's what I'm here for! You take the phone and prep your other patient. You're not alone; we're a team." I realized that nurses are only as good as their team; there will always be times in healthcare when I cannot handle everything myself. If I was proud or refused to work with others, I could have lost a patient that day. My charge nurse was busy, too, but she had the maturity to prioritize needs and the skill to help. I knew I wanted to be like that and not the panicky novice who could not imagine a simple solution to the problem.

That's why seeing all of my co-workers come together for a fundraiser is probably my best work memory. My colleagues helped me personally when I faced struggles, but I felt closer to these nurses than ever before when we served together— and our mutual respect increased exponentially. We stopped suspecting each other of being selfish in work situations and started believing that we could really accomplish great things when we worked together. No one fought for authority or control, but we just offered ourselves, knowing there was nothing that we could do as individuals to ease our friend's burden. It was very humbling. I think that is one of the secrets of being meek: People who are meek count on exponential miracles. I've heard meekness defined as power under control, and I think it must be God's power expressed in our clay-pot faith. Children don't go to their parents with a plan or solution to carry out; they just bring their problems and trust that their parents will figure it out.

When I was a kid, we used to go swimming with my grandparents and play a game called "whirlpool." To play the game, we all swam in the same direction around the pool until it created a current. If one of us turned suddenly in the current, it would pick that person up and carry them away; if we all turned at the same time, we could turn the current. Pride tries to turn and fight the current alone; meekness joins with others to change the current. We all fought our selfishness together that day and became a more generous, loving team with a host of great memories, laughing, and encouraging each other doing something worthwhile. Speaking of inheriting riches, I also found out that day that a lot of my co-workers were Christians. I realized that they didn't choose to be ICU nurses for the money but because they wanted to help people. I think that is why we all heard the call from God to give and serve Joy at that moment. Sometimes I make the wrong assumption that I am alone, and I feel fearful of giving to others in case there might not be enough for me. But I found that I am never alone, and there is always enough in Christ.

Discussion Questions:

For Individuals or Groups

- What do you believe about the people you work with? What is a need in your workplace that you can pray for right now?

- Read Luke 15:25-32 about the prodigal son's brother. Have you ever felt like you were getting cheated in following the Lord? What do you think it means when the father says, "all that is mine is yours" (v. 31)?

Four

CHILDREN OF GOD

"'Truly, I say to you, unless you turn and become like children, you will never enter the kingdom of heaven.'" (Mat. 18:3)

I was helping my grandparents with some spring cleaning, hauling out old Guideposts magazines and Our Daily Bread devotionals, dusting furniture, replacing salt in the water softener, and tending the potted plants, when my grandma said that she needed to step away to put some cookies on a plate. She joked that I needed some "nourishment" after all my hard work. This term for candy and cookies was as old as me because my brother and I used to refuse to leave Grandpa and Grandma's house without candy in our mouths, stating that we would never make it home without "some nourishment for the journey." She would laugh at our Oliver Twist impersonations, and her eyes would crinkle as she brought over the glass candy jar. Shaking her finger, she would chide us with mock sternness, saying, "Only one more!"

When I was a student in college, Grandma continued to stock cookies and candies for me when I visited. I did not complain. My grandparents quoted scripture often while feeding me sweets, and I have heard that young Jewish children are given a taste of honey with the first readings of the Torah to give them a tangible memory of the sweet taste of God's law. In my experience, this is a highly effective teaching method.

While Grandma was busy, Grandpa and I sat on the porch and watched birds fly about, energetically singing amidst the blooming trees and flowering bushes that covered the wild bluff behind the house. We were spring cleaning, and nature was bursting with life and playfulness just outside our window.

"That's how I feel, you know," Grandpa said suddenly. I watched him quizzically and waited for him to explain. I'll never forget the look in his eyes, twinkling with so much mischief and joy. "I'm going to tell you a secret." He paused again for effect. "I feel like Spring inside, just like those birds. I feel like running and jumping and climbing trees!" He slapped his knee and grinned back at me with pure delight in his eyes. There was not an ounce of regret, just bubbling mirth. "This body has gotten old and far too sensible, but inside, I'm still a kid." Then he leaned in close and whispered, "But that's a secret, alright? That's a secret about getting old, and now, you know it, too." I grinned back at him while we watched a pair of squirrels chasing and teasing each other. I tried to picture Grandpa climbing a tree, just as Grandma arrived with a plate of cookies.

I was surprised to find, a couple of years later when I went to work at a long-term care facility, that several residents confided exactly the same thing to me: "I'm young inside, it's just that this body has gotten old. Inside I still feel like a child!" I thought it was fascinating that this experience of being a young person in an old body was a seemingly universal experience. I knew these adventurous seniors would be thrilled to get new bodies for climbing trees in heaven.

But then I noticed, too, that not everyone described aging that way; there were always some people who continually talked about how old they were. They felt old both inside and outside—and maybe they always had. I've known young adults who continually talked about how tired and old they felt; I can imagine that attitude could become a lifelong pattern.

When I think about it, our Father in heaven is really old. When I put His ageless seniority and eternal wisdom in perspective with the 90-year-olds and centenarians I've known, they really are just kids. When Jesus tells us to become like children, he's stating the obvious: Act your age and don't pretend to know it all. Listen and obey with enthusiasm because you'll grow up fast. And it does go by fast. Our lives are a breath in the line of eternity—but this childhood on earth shapes our eternal identity, and sometime later, we will get to join the "grown-up table" at the heavenly banquet.

Discussion Questions:

For Individuals or Groups

- Have you ever felt like you were not your age? Are you an old person or a young person inside?

- If you kept your current attitude for eternity, what would you want to change?

Five

NOTHING TO GIVE

"That according to the riches of his glory he may grant you to be strengthened with power through his Spirit in your inner being, so that Christ may dwell in your hearts through faith—that you, being rooted and grounded in love, may have strength to comprehend with all the saints what is the breadth and length and height and depth, and to know the love of Christ that surpasses knowledge, that you may be filled with all the fullness of God." (Eph. 3:16-19)

I had never felt so alone. My husband and son were struggling to keep our small business afloat, and I was four hours away trying to take care of our premature baby in the NICU. Our families were days away and could not stay with us to help—we had no place to keep them. There was a hang-up with my benefits and our account was nearing empty.

My postpartum hormones were swinging low. So many people reached out to us, but I still spent most of the day alone and worried.

I was scared of the emotions I felt at that time, and I didn't want to act how I felt. I wanted to be ruled by the Lord and how He wanted me to live, but I also knew I had zero strength to make it alone. I knelt tearfully to pray, and I felt the Lord asking me if anyone had it as bad as me. Well, of course—it could always be worse, right? But that wasn't much comfort to me. Then I sensed Him leading me to find someone who "had it worse" than me and serve them. Basically, God was showing me how damaging it is to my spirit to think only of my problems and myself. My tears stopped, and I knew He was right. I believed He was leading me to do something for someone else, and it would be the best medicine to lift my spirit.

The only problem is that I felt I had nothing to give. I felt I did not have enough time, money, care, or love for my own family, much less to give to another. I was drained to empty and already felt like a failure. How could I add more, only to fail at it? I asked God to help me think of something I could do. What could someone do with nothing but problems to offer?

Later that day, I was scrolling through messages and was interested to read another update on a couple from church: Victor had just returned from serving in the military in Afghanistan to discover that he had a brain tumor. The prognosis was that it would most likely be terminal, but he was going for palliative brain surgery next week. I knew that in his situation there was not much that anyone could do at this point but pray. A light bulb turned on: I can pray. It was the only gift I could give, but it was a good one.

Suddenly, the ideas started flowing. I messaged a friend in church—one of the saints that I highly respected, who would surely tell me gently if my decisions were flawed—and asked if we could put together a prayer meeting for Victor, and could her quilting group make a prayer quilt with our written prayers all over it. She thought it was a great idea. She enlisted her son-in-law to host, coordinated volunteers to bake and cook and serve, made plans for how to put written prayers on fabric, and worked with me, and with Victor's family, to set a date.

Tons of church members showed up to pray. We all wrote prayers on brightly colored quilt squares, entered notes of encouragement in a journal, ate delicious snacks, and then squeezed together in that living room, some in chairs, some on the floor, to pray. We prayed that Victor would be miraculously healed, that he and his family would be comforted by God's Presence, and many other blessings. I felt so connected to God's people. I felt "filled to the measure" with God's love.

We watched and prayed the day of his surgery, checking updates throughout the day and night. He got out of surgery, but they hadn't been able to take out as much of the tumor as they had wanted. Then, he was rushed back when his nurse found evidence that he was bleeding. We prayed harder. They took out more of the tumor and stabilized the bleeding. We breathed a sigh of relief and continued to pray. The neurosurgeon was already saying that he was a miracle.

Today, everyone agrees that Victor's story is a miracle. Years later, he died and went home to be with His Lord, but those extra years he spent with his wife, seeing their son grow up together, was a beautiful testimony that he shared at every opportunity, glorifying God for his recovery. I would have felt happy for them when I heard the good news, but I felt so much more invested after being part of a prayer meeting that agreed in faith for his healing. I got to see God's power at work in miraculous ways while I waited for His answer to my own trials.

Speaking of those trials, my premature baby is now in elementary school and is tall for her age. She is healthy and beautiful and loves books. It was a difficult time, but God provided for us in every way and through many miracles. My faith is much bigger now after witnessing His glorious riches—first in other people's lives and later in ours. I guess that's why the Scripture says that we will overcome by the blood of the Lamb and the word of our testimony (Rev. 12:11). It is so encouraging to take part in other people's lives and problems and to see God answer with power. That is how I grasped how wide and long and high and deep is the love of Christ (Eph 3:18).

Discussion Questions:

For Individuals or Groups

- What is a testimony that has encouraged you recently? Have you tried asking anyone about how God is working in their lives?

- Have you ever seen God provide for a need miraculously? If so, were you surprised?

Six

SPA CHALLENGE

"Love one another with brotherly affection. Outdo one another in showing honor." (Rom. 12:10)

It all started with my preceptor in the ICU. One of my first days on the unit, she explained that ICU nurses do "total care" for their patients because they are in a more fragile condition. "We don't have any nurse assistants here because anytime you turn your patient, they could code. Besides," she paused "it gives us a chance to go the extra mile to help someone feel better. I've shaved legs, trimmed beards, braided hair, and done make-up for my patients. Sometimes people just feel better when they get spruced up. Plus, it's kind of a running competition for the nursing team—we try to outdo each other." She smiled confidently, winked, and pulled a set of brand new, high-quality razors, shaving cream, make-up samples, and hair-ties from her locker. "The stuff the hospital provides is not that great, so I bring new packages of goodies that I can share with patients when there's time. If you need any of this for your patient, just let me know, and it's yours."

The challenge was on.

My next night shift, I started to set-up for a patient bath when I suddenly stopped to think, "What could I do to make this an extra-special bath?" I wanted to be like my preceptor. I wanted to outdo her kindness (and she set a high standard!). I grabbed shaving cream and a razor, lotion, extra pillows, and a plastic tweezer that I thought I could use to clean under my patient's nails. I got to work with a smile and talked my patient through every step. By the time I was shaving his stubble and cleaning under his nails he started crying and praying out loud, "Gracias a Dios! Gracias a Dios!" (Thank you, God!)

I was floored. I took his hand in mine and said, "Sí, gracias a Dios por todos" (yes, thanks to God for everything).

He hollered again, "Ah, and God has sent me an angel who believes in You! Thank you, God! Thank you!" He wiped his eyes and said, "It is much better, now. Much better."

We really didn't talk anymore. He was all choked up and so was I.

That night didn't even begin to compare with other "Spa Challenges" that my colleagues had completed for their patients. It didn't even make mention on the scoreboard. There was no pedicure, and my haircutting and beard trimming skills were sub-par. But kindness speaks volumes. I had to stop and wonder why it took a friendly competition to make me try a little harder to be creative in kindness. I had to wonder why this didn't happen more often. I turned to scripture and thanked God for sending an example to me in real life through my preceptor.

When the Good Samaritan stopped to help a hurting man, that man had been stripped, beaten, and left for dead. Jesus was stripped, beaten and left for dead as well, but He instructed his followers to love others without bias. But unless we allow the Holy Spirit to search our souls, we do not "naturally" reach out to strangers with kindness, and we never love our enemies. The Bible says, "You shall love the Lord your God with all your heart and with all your soul and with all your might" (Deut. 6:5). That means I have a heart, soul, and body that I can love with.

I will probably need to spend the rest of my life in this endeavor to love God with all three parts of myself, to the degree that He deserves, rather than according to what I'm capable of offering. But I can also say that it has changed the way I treat other people. When I look at other people, I now see three parts that are made to love God. I am called, just like the Good Samaritan, to love all three parts. I am called to serve their physical, emotional, and spiritual needs holistically.

I've learned now that it's not just the manicure that makes a "Spa Challenge" bath so much better; it's the time spent together, respecting the whole person while discussing thoughts and fears, and coming with joy to feed the soul. I'm thankful to my nurse preceptor for challenging me to slow down and spend some time really caring for my patients and for highlighting why every human being is precious.

Discussion Questions:

For Individuals or Groups

- Have you ever had a "spa moment," where you felt clean, calm, and relaxed? What is your favorite spa treat?

- What are some things that are missing in the hospital environment that help people feel a lot better? Is there any way to improve that?

Seven

PRAYING WITH THE VP

"**P**raying at all times in the Spirit, with all prayer and supplication. To that end keep alert with all perseverance, making supplication for all the saints, and also for me, that words may be given to me in opening my mouth boldly to proclaim the mystery of the gospel" (Eph. 6:18-19)

I sat with my co-worker, Valorie, in the lunchroom. We were talking about how God was convicting us to pray for the hospital's leadership. They were all heading out on a business trip to give a response to internal problems and share their vision for the future. We felt like they were good leaders who cared about the hospital, but we felt for some reason like they might need some heavenly help in this meeting. For the first time ever, I looked my co-worker in the eye and said, "We need to pray for our Vice President."

Her eyes got wide, and she sat back a little; she looked utterly stunned. When she found her words, she looked up and said, "Alright, then. Thank You, Lord, for confirming Your voice through many witnesses!" She laughed nervously.

"Huh?" I was confused.

"I just sensed the Lord telling me to go to her office and offer to pray for her. Now. You just confirmed that it's from Him!"

We stared at each other in awkward silence.

Our VP, Athena, was an animated leader who was known for firing people on the spot. Anytime I spoke with Athena, I feared for my job; she ruled like a Medici, strategic and full of surprises. She sometimes mentioned stuff about having an eternal purpose, but I had no idea what her personal beliefs were, and we both realized that we may not still have jobs by the time we left her office. Maybe we would get a security escort out the door? Or perhaps God saw her needs, and there was a reason we needed to pray with her right away.

"There's no backing out of it now, is there?" Valorie asked timidly.

Valorie was never timid. She was bold and brave and said what she wanted. But she was scared now.

"Let's go to our office and pray privately. Then we'll go together. You know what it says about 'two or three gathered together in My Name.' There must be a reason why she needs prayer now."

"Okay, it's a deal," she agreed.

We quickly packed up our lunches and retreated to the

office. We did not pray long. It seemed simple: Let us obey You and do the right thing, and if You see fit to let us keep our jobs, great. If not, then we trust You. "Most of all, please open Athena's heart to You, Lord. Help her to know You like we do."

Still nervous, we swished water to clean our teeth, straightened our clothes and hair, and hoped we would not be thrown out on our ears. When we knocked on the side of Athena's open door to let her know we were there, there was an awkward pause when she looked up. "Oh, my goodness— what is it?" Athena asked. "You guys look like you're going to tell me something terrible!"

We laughed nervously and Valorie cleared her throat, and started speaking rapidly, "We just wanted to ask if you would like us to pray for you before your business trip. We know that it's important, and we just wanted to pray for favor and safety for your trip."

There was a long pause. My hands started sweating.

"I'm really happy you came to me like this," Athena said, completely serious.

Valorie looked at me; I looked at Valorie. Did that mean she was glad it would be easy to fire us both at once? Or that she actually wanted to pray?

Athena continued, "I've been reading a lot by this Christian author, and I feel like there's a lot of growth that needs to happen on the inside of me. While part of me is concerned that my plane is going to crash, and God sent you to warn me—" she laughed again, "the other part of me is just really pleased that you would cross the 'power barrier' to reach out to me and help me be closer to God." She nodded and reached out her hands, "I would love it if you would pray for me."

We prayed a short prayer of blessing, favor, and safe travels, and then we left quietly. As we turned to leave, she looked us each in the eye and said, "Thank you, it really means a lot."

Discussion Questions:

For Individuals or Groups

- Why is it so hard to pray with someone when you are unsure how they will feel about it?

- What are some prayers that have been answered when you overcame your fear?

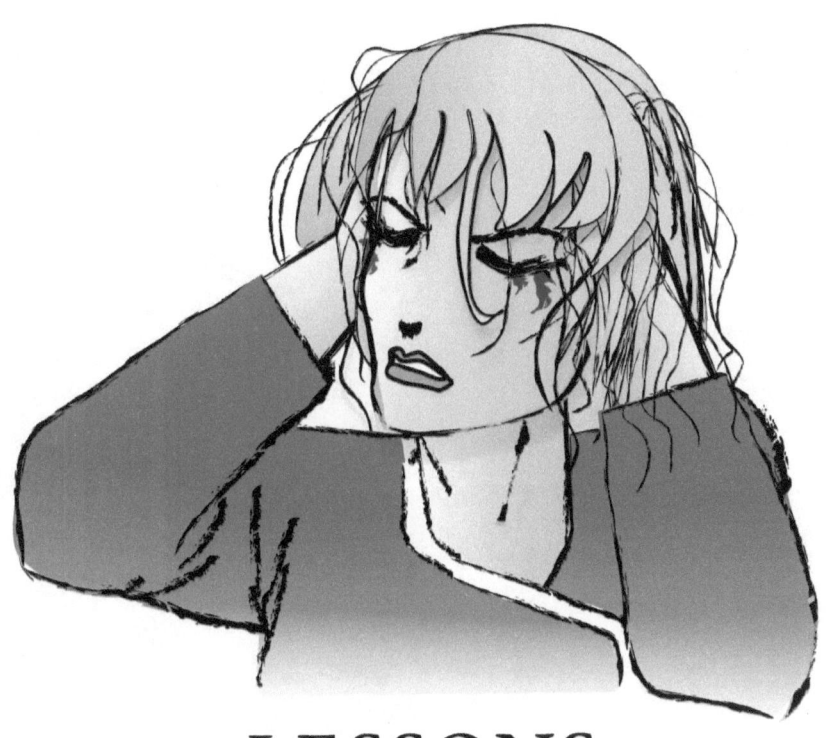

LESSONS
(SILLY & SERIOUS)

These stories are object lessons from my
experiences

One

TREAT MY PAIN

"The God who made the world and everything in it, being Lord of heaven and earth, does not live in temples made by man, nor is He served by human hands, as though He needed anything, since He Himself gives to all mankind life and breath and everything." (Acts 17:24-25)

My husband was folded over the motel toilet, ashen and sweating. He told me between gasps that there was a fierce, sharp pain in his flank and that it hurt in his lower back when he urinated. We were on a mission trip to canvas neighborhoods with invitations to a Gospel presentation. Earlier that day, we went "door-to-door" in run-down neighborhoods with slapstick homes that looked ready to fall off their cement block foundations. Each door was at the end of a chain-link fence filled with hungry dogs that often escaped and chased us in the 100-degree humid heat. In the naïveté of early parenthood, we had decided that having a baby would not prevent us from serving in the church's mission, and we now found ourselves running from wild dogs in 100-degree heat with an infant in a stroller. Yeah, not the brightest thing we ever did—and we had only consumed soda for most of the day as that was all that was available. Now, as my husband moaned on the motel room floor, the result appeared to be an excruciating kidney stone.

I assured my husband that this condition would not kill him, that the nausea and vomiting was probably due to the pain he was feeling, and since he didn't have a fever, he would likely be okay, as long as he flushed the stone out with plenty of water.

My husband said, "I think you should take me to the hospital."

"Here? I don't even know where the hospital is, and our son is sound asleep—I don't think we should expose our baby to all those hospital germs." My husband is a strong, rational man, and I knew he would want to use our resources wisely and not risk harm to our child. "Besides, they won't remove the kidney stone or anything like that—they will only treat your pain and send you home. I think we should just stay here and push fluids."

My husband swung around and reached for me, disheveled, gray-faced, and sweating, "Treat my pain!" he bellowed.

I grimaced and nodded, shaken. "Okay, okay. I'll take you to the hospital."

Our pastor's wife was kind enough to stay in our room while our baby slept, and the pastor came with us in our car to make sure we were safe. I drove, terrified, through the dark city, hoping that I would not accidentally drive into Mexico in the middle of the night or run over one of the fierce, wild dogs that roamed the city. At one point, I lost my bearings and pulled over to the curb on a side street, so I could check the map on my phone. My husband glanced nervously out the window from a reclined position in the back seat, still groaning in pain.

"Ah, we need to move now," he called up to me.

"I know it hurts, but I just need to find which way to turn," I answered, fretting at the map on my phone.

"Move now! There is a gang coming for us, and they are almost here."

I looked up and saw about fifteen men emerging from the shadows across the street, and they were walking toward us with a swagger of set jaws and ready fists. At two o'clock in the morning, I assumed it was not the men's prayer breakfast. I looked around quickly to make sure I was still clear and hit the gas. We looped through sketchy neighborhoods with broken roads full of potholes until we found our way back to the highway and saw the red "Emergency Room" sign ahead. It was God's grace alone that got us there because I was utterly lost at that point.

My husband hobbled in and when the ED nurse saw him looking scruffy and wincing in pain, he must have thought he was a drug-seeker. I have to say, my husband kind of looked the part as an otherwise healthy-looking young male.

However, they gave him IV anti-nausea medication and a half-dose of non-opioid Toradol, and my exhausted husband disproved all suspicion that he was just there to seek opioids: In about one minute, he lay face-down on the cot, completely knocked out and drooling. The poor guy!

"Ah, I see he won't need any more pain medication then," the night nurse chuckled.

I asked about payment, and they sent someone from accounting to help answer my questions. It turned out that it would cost exactly the same amount to pay with or without insurance—insurance would be charged at a higher rate, so our copay would be the same as the cash rate even if our insurance did not cover the visit at all. So much for conserving our resources.

We drove home early after a short nap, armed with prescriptions and plenty of water, and laughed about the previous night's conversation where I had completely ignored my husband's top priority—his fifth vital sign, no less. He quickly forgave me since I braved gangsters in the middle of the night to get him some relief. But I realized that it's frighteningly easy to look at problems with a desire to fix them, rather than seeing the person and their need for comfort. I appreciate that Jesus displayed both a solution to problems as well as compassion. In fact, He took time to listen to people's problems even though He already knew what they were, and He definitely could have interrupted for the sake of efficiency. I also felt grateful that my husband interrupted my analysis to tell me what he needed, but as a young nurse I filed a memory that I needed to listen more and try to empathize because my patients may not feel comfortable interrupting my analytics to tell me how they feel. If I did not make it a priority, things like pain could just get lost in the shuffle even though it's a treatable problem.

Then I wondered, what about the people whose pain cannot be treated, and they are not safe (from gangsters, for example)? I hear stories all the time of people who are never safe or well-fed, yet their faith is strong, and their optimism is influential. I love getting newsletters from The Voice of the Martyrs because they share true stories and testimonies of people who are going through a lot more than me and have sustained faith in Jesus. I can learn a lot from those stories, remembering that my material needs are secondary, and faith is stronger than persecution. Sometimes I think studying the Bible is inconvenient, but many Christians around the world are not able to read the Bible, so they memorize entire chapters and devour audio Bibles, studying even when it's illegal to do so.

In contrast, our worldly perspective puts physical needs first. Most Americans believe they cannot and should not address spiritual needs until they have achieved health and safety, whatever that means for them. And how can someone ever be safe from death since we are all mortal? When Maslow's hierarchy of needs was introduced in the field of psychology, he wrote about universal needs among human beings and then assigned priorities in a pyramid shape. Maslow said that the lower, broad tiers of the pyramid included basic human needs such as physical safety and survival, and he presented the opinion that these needs must take priority, and even be satisfied, before an individual could develop their mind and spirit.[1]

When I read "the faith chapter" in the Bible (Heb. 11), I cannot help but notice that none of these heroes of the faith would be able to get past the first tier of Maslow's hierarchy of needs, yet they somehow emerged fearless and faithful. In contrast, I witnessed Maslow's beliefs shape generations of people as they pushed for better health and fitness in defiance of their mortality and to the detriment of their spiritual health. So many people complained to us that they had "done everything right" with their health, and yet here they were, facing heart disease at age sixty-eight. Did they really think that their bodies were invincible because they went jogging every day and ate broccoli?

As a Christian, I know that I could run marathons but struggle to pray. I could grow my own organic vegetables and still not be able to sleep at night. I could be well-fed and safe, but my body would always crave more from the God-shaped hole of loneliness and fear without Him. While stewardship of my body is a worthy pursuit, I realized that I could never accomplish the goal of complete physical safety, or achieve health that counteracted my mortality. If Maslow was correct and physical health was a prerequisite to spiritual health, then I would never become mature in my mind and soul. After spending time at the bedside of hundreds of people listening to their needs, I kind of think Maslow's pyramid is like those ancient pyramids found buried within mountains of dirt and decay: Most ancient pyramids were found by climbing to the

---

1 Potter, PA; Perry, AG (2005). Fundamentals of Nursing (6th edition, p. 93). Elsevier.

top and discovering that there are shaped stones underneath all the dirt, or by flying overhead to peer through a dense rainforest of tree tops—in other words, they are lost until someone can get a higher perspective and see the top of the pyramid. In the same way, Maslow had his priorities upside down. We'll never be content having our physical needs met if our spiritual needs are unfulfilled. After all the physical troubles I've had, I'm certainly not going to wait on my body to be pain-free before I get my spiritual life in better shape.

Pain is a signal that warns us when something is wrong in our bodies—but it is also a physical signal to our souls reminding us of our mortality. We are supposed to remember that this body is temporary; pain reminds us that we will die someday, and it repeatedly presents itself through our nervous system. You can see the mortal alarm ringing every time a small child scrapes their knee on the sidewalk, and they completely panic at the sight of blood. One of the first things their parents tell them is, "It's going to be okay; you're not dying." When we treat pain, it allows us a chance to find the physical cause, but it also helps us consider our eternity. Every stubbed toe and skinned knee is an opportunity to thank God for our next breath and get right with Him before our lives are over. And what is it about the sight of blood anyway? The Bible describes a bloody Lamb taking the judgment seat in heaven, and I wonder if we just hate to be reminded of the wounds inflicted on Him for our sins?

I have found that it's crucial to preach the Gospel when I go to help with any physical need—whether in caregiving, financial support, or any other type of practical ministry. Even if someone is antagonistic to the Gospel, I always ask them if they would like me to pray with them, and they nearly always give permission with gratitude. Offering prayer is a great chance to stop and listen well—it's the chance for someone to say, "I have pain," and point to the physical, emotional, or spiritual suffering that hurts most. I would say that Maslow's pyramid is structurally unsound; I certainly do not count on physical health to make me "my best self." No, I will not be worshipping at the pyramid-temple of Maslow; I worship the living God who does not dwell in temples made with hands (Acts 17:24), and whose healing power touches not just our aching bodies, but our sinful souls as well.

Discussion Questions:

For Individuals or Groups

- Have you ever gotten caught up in physical fitness or seeking comfort and safety before addressing spiritual health? How do you prioritize your soul today?

- Did you ever feel that it was not helpful to talk to someone about spiritual things when you were serving them? Why or why not?

Two

DIFFICULT QUESTIONS

"If in Christ we have hope in this life only, we are of all people most to be pitied." (1Cor. 15:19)

From my earliest time in nursing school, sources like *Potter and Perry's Fundamentals of Nursing* explained, "as nurses, it becomes important to accept and acknowledge others' beliefs and not spend work time trying to convert others to our personal beliefs."[1] Sure, coercion is wrong, but one of the core beliefs of Christianity is sharing the good news of Jesus with others. What is a Christian to do when they are told to leave their faith at the door when they come to work? Is it ethical to watch someone die in their sins when you know the One who can set them free? I felt so conflicted and unsure. So I looked for answers from Christian sources.

1 Potter, PA; Perry, AG (2005). Fundamentals of Nursing (6th edition, p. 550). Elsevier.

One article started with a warning story of how a nurse was placed on a leave of absence after asking a patient if there was anything the patient would like her to pray about. The undertone was that any mention of faith or spiritual matters could get you in trouble, and it is probably "more ethical" to remain silent. Another story relayed how a nurse was fired for simply talking about the afterlife, without making value judgments, because it offended the family to overhear the conversation. Their recommendation was the same as the secular's: leave Christ outside the hospital doors, as His name might be offensive.

Offensive? Nurses do a lot of things that are offensive. Besides working with body fluids, I have even found that some patients find bathing an offensive practice, but it does not keep us from preaching the good news of germ removal because they will undoubtedly find it helpful as they fight infection. So why is spiritual care so taboo?

And it's not like people who are sick and dying don't have spiritual concerns. I've been asked some hard, spiritual questions in my role as a nurse. Everyone from co-workers to patient families have asked me questions like:

- "Do you think God can ever forgive me?"
- "Do you think she is possessed? She wasn't like this before she was abused, and all the physical tests are negative."
- "What are you going to do to make sure I don't die? I'm so afraid."
- "What will happen to her when she dies?"

- "Do you think God is punishing me?"

At the bedside, I usually offered to have a chaplain see the patient when they had questions about chronic illness, coping, and dying. There were a lot of questions I simply could not answer. But when I called the chaplain, something funny happened: While the patient was happy to have someone to talk to, and it was developmentally appropriate to discuss spiritual matters, sometimes the family became upset, saying, "Oh, he doesn't want that. He's not going to die." I also found that my nurse peers would often raise their eyebrows when they saw a note in the Kardex that a chaplain was requested. "They're not dying, are they? Why would you ask for a chaplain?" Why does everyone think that spiritual care should only occur the moment before we die?

Even Potter & Perry say that avoiding the subject of mortality entirely doesn't really help advocate for healthy coping with illness. [2] Developmentally, there is a stage of life where we all need to prepare for death. It's a time of looking at our legacy with satisfaction or regret and taking care of relationships and business before we die. If the patient is ready to discuss the afterlife already, developmentally, why would we halt their progress because it's uncomfortable for us? While I privately prayed for all my patients, I cannot say that I fully understood the responsibility I had as I sat with the most vulnerable people in the world: Human beings who were running out of time. But of all the times and places I have experienced in my Christian life, I haven't sensed the

2 Potter, PA; Perry, AG (2005). Fundamentals of Nursing (6th edition, p. 573). Elsevier.

potential for persecution for my faith as acutely as when a patient would ask me about spiritual things.

One patient that made me struggle with this responsibility was a man named Amos, who was covered with sores that oozed and caused him continuous pain. He had a particularly virulent skin infection. Every time I walked in the room, I was overwhelmed by his suffering, by the heat of our isolation gear, and by the odor of his wounds. Amos was homeless; he had no family, and when he developed sores on his legs, he covered them with trash bags on the street. They became infected and festered with odorous, purulent fluid so that just walking into his room made me gag. He itched constantly, and his wounds caused him constant pain. When I entered his room, I wore two masks and put menthol under my nose to keep myself from retching because the odor was so terrible. And he could never leave that odor because it was all over him. His condition tore at my heart.

He started making comments to the nurses about being afraid of dying, while at the same time longing for an end to his suffering. I knew I should start a conversation with him, but it was so challenging to go into his room, and frankly nauseating to stay with him for any amount of time. I found myself avoiding any discussion. I was also working with a different crew than I usually worked with. I thought, "Tomorrow, I'll talk to him tomorrow. If this group of nurses hear that I've talked with him about spiritual things, they'll give me trouble."

The next night, I discovered that he had checked out against medical advice to "die on the street where he won't bother anyone." I wept. I had a dream that night about the rich man and Lazarus from the Bible (Luke 16), and the question posed to me by the Holy Spirit was, "If Lazarus suffered all his life, is it not better that he received relief in heaven, rather than suffer for eternity as well?" What if Amos never received relief in either life? I was crushed in my spirit and began to repent and pray for his salvation, asking God to send someone that would care for him wherever he was. I had cared more for my physical comfort and reputation among peers than for this poor man's eternal state. I wish I had a nice, tidy resolution where I could say that Amos became a Christian and found relief in heaven, but I don't know anything about what happened to him after that night. I had no idea it would be my last chance, and I never saw a resolution to the suffering he went through.

Another time, I had gotten to know a man named John after helping him when he coded. He had developed septic shock on the unit, and I had been called to coach the nurses and collaborate with his physician on our brand-new septic shock protocol. Every time I saw him, I felt proud of the new protocol our hospital had implemented: One moment he was confused with crashing vital signs, and the next moment he was wide-awake and asking for lunch.

John had terminal lung cancer, but I found out from his nurse that his family had asked for some time before they told him. I got to know him on my rounds because I was charged with the task of assessing every central line on the unit daily. I had a nine-to-five office job now and enjoyed this brief chance to interact with patients at the bedside again. I did not have the impression from our talks that he knew God, but it seemed that his brush with death during that code had caused him to consider how he felt about dying. He adamantly told me that he wanted to live to be part of his grandchildren's lives. He adored each of them and showed me pictures, telling me stories of their budding skills and interests. He said he would fight to get better, so he could continue spending time with them. Later, I got to visit with his son, and we all got to know each other well.

One Friday, my husband asked if I could please hurry home and try to leave early. I had worked some evenings earlier in the week to speak at board meetings, and he simply wanted to reclaim some time together. I had not finished my work as quickly as I had hoped due to other codes that day. However, as I entered the unit to check central lines at about 4:45pm, the nurse told me that they had all met today and shared John's prognosis with him. He had decided to become a DNR/DNI code status.

When I saw him, John was breathless and a bit tearful. He brightened when I came in, and we chatted a bit about his family. He invited me to take a seat, as we had done before, to stay with him and talk. I apologized and asked if we could catch up next time because I was running late today. "My husband misses me, and I think that's a good thing." I winked. "So, I should probably get going today."

He smiled, patted my hand, and told me to run home to my precious family. "You're making the right choice because they won't be with you forever, and each moment with the people you love is so precious. My son will be here soon, so we will both spend some time with our families today." He winked back, and we said a warm goodbye.

I didn't know it would be our last goodbye: He died that night with his son at the bedside. At first, it was like a knife twisted in my heart, knowing that I missed the opportunity to ask if there was anything he needed to do to be ready, but when my Christian colleague saw the distress on my face, she quickly added, "It's okay, I sat with John. I was there. We talked a great deal, and I phoned his sister, so he could tell her he forgave her." I am still learning to watch for the opportunity to love someone who may not be there tomorrow. Psalm 103:15 says, "As for man, his days are like grass; he flourishes like a flower of the field; for the wind passes over it, and it is gone, and its place knows it no more." I am bound by the limits of time and schedules, but God is not limited by time. Can you imagine the pressure if I was the only person in the world who could "save" a man?

In the case of John, I found out later that another believer was there to talk with him about his life after death. While my colleague's kindness did not make me feel better about leaving John on his last day, it does assure me that God is bigger than my failures. I treasure my Christian colleagues, and I remember their names today because I know that God's people always show up when they are needed. God never misses a divine appointment. The God who began a good work in me is faithful to complete it (Phil. 1:6). I thank God for His faithfulness and for continuing to teach me.

Another teaching moment was when Jewel asked for prayer. She was a friendly, attractive young woman who worked at the hospital coffee stand. She was always joking with people, and I noticed that she made a special effort to learn everyone's names. She was always laughing about something, and we all loved talking to her. So when another co-worker sent out a text, "Anyone who is available, we are meeting to pray for Jewel right now," we gathered quickly to support our friend. I had no idea what was going on, but when Jewel walked into the room, I knew something was seriously wrong. She was crying and trying so hard to be strong and stay composed for work. She was devastated by a personal loss that she never saw coming. We prayed with her, but I really didn't know how to pray and honestly did a poor job of it, struggling to find words and rambling on too long. We encouraged her and grieved her loss, but it was a hard time, and Jewel didn't want to talk anymore about it; suddenly, she was quiet and pale, and while she told us she was fine, she didn't look fine at all. I continued to pray for her, more for safety and recovery than with much faith.

When I went to get a cup of coffee a few days later, Jewel was absolutely beaming. The coffee stand was packed with a mid-day coffee rush, but Jewel greeted me warmly and started sharing an update to her story. She could not contain sharing her testimony with me, even as the line of people forming behind me got longer:

"I was so broken, you know? But I saw this online sermon the other day, and it was just like you ladies had said. He talked about belonging to God's family and letting God finish your story. It just really resonated with me that there's more. There is something better. This is not the end of my story.

"I cried out to God right then and said, 'I NEED YOU, GOD!' I was so desperate. Immediately, I felt this heavy, warm Presence. It was like He was holding me and hugging me, and the tears just poured out of me. I felt His love! I have so much joy just bubbling out of me now! I want nothing else than to be with Him, and I am so grateful for your prayers. I am so thankful for Jesus!"

I was stunned and kind of embarrassed: I felt so honored to have my pathetic prayers added to the testimony she was sharing—it was really, really humbling. But all I had done was pray a pathetic, generic prayer for "comfort," and even that was done poorly. It's like when you drive down the street on a beautiful day, but you're so distracted or focused on something else that you don't even notice the beauty all around you: God was working, but I didn't even look up or notice.

So while I long for closure to all of these stories—to know that both John and Amos are in heaven now—I have to resist the urge to soak in shame or pity over my missed opportunities. My spiritual sensitivity is increasing with each hard lesson—as long as I listen to the Teacher. I don't get to know what God knows, and I am not perfect like Him. That's good to remember. I have to listen to Him if I'm going to pick up on those divine appointments. But He is perfect, and knowing that "everyone who calls on the name of the LORD shall be saved" (Joel 2:32) is an incredible relief for an imperfect messenger.

Discussion Questions:

For Individuals or Groups

- Do you tend to be slow to respond to the Lord's direction? How can you improve? What opportunities do you believe you may have missed?

- What opportunities are available to you now? Pray for anyone that comes to mind and ask God to give you courage and sensitivity to His leading.

Three

COLANDER

"**A**nd Jesus, looking at him, loved him, and said to him, 'You lack one thing...'" (Mark 10:21a)

I woke up at dawn, and it was still cool and dark all over the house. I put on a robe and slippers and crept out of my room to see what had awakened me. I met my older brother at the stairs, and we looked at each other knowingly as we heard the recliner upstairs fold back. As we turned the corner at the top of the stairs, we saw a familiar scene: My mother was reclined in a chair with an ice pack on her head and a bowl on the table beside her. She suffered from migraines, and when the pain was really bad, she felt horribly nauseous. Usually, the only thing that would cure the nausea was pizza (don't judge). You could try giving her broth and crackers, but it wouldn't help. Pizza, however, did the trick every time.

But now—in the pre-dawn hours—there was no pizza, and she was suffering with pain, nausea, and light-sensitivity. We offered to fix something for her to eat, or fetch her some medicine, but she said she would be fine with just a cup of coffee for now. Her hand held an ice pack to her forehead, and she didn't look at us, but her voice was strong. She reached over, still holding the ice pack on her head, and held up the bowl she had grabbed in case she needed to vomit. I guess that was supposed to let us know she was okay.

I stared at my brother. He stared at me. Then we started to laugh.

Confused, my mom uncovered one of her eyes to look questioningly at us. "What?" she asked, getting irritated with our noise and lack of empathy.

"Mom," my brother began, "I'm relieved that you thought to set a colander next to you in case you should need to vomit, but..." He paused for effect.

Her eyes widened, and the ice pack came down as she stared, open-mouthed at the colander in her hands. "It was dark... I couldn't see well...they're all stacked in the same place," she sputtered. Then we all laughed and laughed until her head hurt, and she needed to put the ice pack back on her forehead. We made breakfast and gave her some coffee, asking jovially if she would like us to pour it through the colander before serving it. She never lived that one down. How many times have I been absolutely convinced that I am prepared—dressed and ready—but I have actually missed the most obvious part?

One of my first "colander" moments as a nurse was when

I noticed that my patient's breathing was speeding up, and they looked "off" somehow. She was a new admission, and I took a set of vital signs, repositioned her with the head of the bed elevated, paged the doctor and the respiratory therapist, and looked up the patient's medication list for any available interventions. I asked my mentor if there was anything else I should do, and she said I should make sure I have the chart ready to write down the doctor's orders. Done. I was ready.

The physician called back, and I began explaining that the patient was breathing poorly, shared the vital signs and let him know that albuterol had not resolved the rapid breathing. "What do her lungs sound like?" he asked.

My scalp tensed and a prickly sensation rushed down my arms and legs. My face flushed.

"Hello? What were her lung sounds?" he repeated politely.

"Let me just go check, if you'll please hold one moment" I said, crossing my fingers.

I could feel his incredulous response. There was a breath-less pause—just long enough for my face to flush even redder, as I felt my pulse begin to pound in my forehead.

Then it began.

"WHAT ARE YOU DOING CALLING ME WITHOUT CHECKING THE LUNG SOUNDS!!!! Do you think I can just tell over the phone? Oh, by this ring it must be PNEUMONIA! Oh wait, when my cell vibrated it sounded more like an embolus. What are you [bleeping] doing paging me about respiratory distress without listening to the patient's lungs!?"

I waited there, taking deep breaths, absorbing all the hatred emanating from a poorly informed late-night page. I covered the phone and asked the charge nurse, who was staring at me now because the yelling could be heard over the phone and asked if she would please listen to 218A's lung sounds for me. She nodded, left quickly, and returned with a slip of paper stating, "consolidated bases, soft crackles above."

I whispered an ashamed "thank you" to my charge nurse and, when the doctor paused for a ragged breath, I apologized and shared this information. He ordered a chest x-ray, as needed oxygen, and some medication. Then he asked me to call with the results of the x-ray, still muttering under his breath about the incompetence of nurses these days.

The patient stabilized with a new aerosol medication, and antibiotics were started for community-acquired pneumonia. I never forgot to do a focused assessment for any change in my patient's condition after that shaming experience. I knew the doctor was right. Even though my pride was indignant about being coarsely yelled at like a poorly behaved dog, I knew that it was not the time to be proud when a patient was unstable and needed my help. My charge nurse asked if I was okay, and I said I was fine and had learned an important lesson. She nodded and said that all nurses learn those lessons but that I should keep it up, I was doing just fine. I was just grateful that the patient recovered so well.

I think lots of people felt that way when Jesus came—that mixture of humiliated pride and desire for truth and purpose.

The rich young ruler had prepared well—he carefully followed Jewish law and planned a purposeful appearance on the path where Jesus was going to travel. He even had an introductory speech prepared. He was ready to receive his reward that very day. Jesus tells him that no one is good (Mark 10:18). But this young man has an answer for that: He has followed all the rules for his entire life. Jesus loves him (and does not correct his statement), and says he lacks only one thing (Mark 10:21). The young man was not prepared for that! Maybe he wanted to defend himself, or maybe he wondered how he could have missed something so obvious. Either way, the Bible says he went away discouraged, and it sparks a crucial conversation with the disciples about salvation.

It's so easy to get defensive. I want everyone to think I am the best Christian, the best wife and mother, the best nurse— but I am just dust, and a single conversation with the Lord blows me away like powder in the wind (Psalm 103). When I hold back from defending myself, and receive correction, I can learn something valuable about being truly prepared.

Discussion Questions:

For Individuals or Groups

- What do you believe you are poorly prepared for? Have you received correction or warning about something that would help you prepare better? Pray and ask for God's help.

- What do you feel well-prepared for? Take time to humbly give your plans to God and ask Him to take charge of the matter.

Four

GERMS

"And by these you shall become unclean. Whoever touches their carcass shall be unclean until the evening." (Lev. 11:24)

I could say so much about germs. As a sepsis coordinator, people used to see me in the hallway and greet me, "Hey, I saw an infection and thought of you!" Then they would share every detail about the most interesting and noteworthy infections they had seen that week. These were the stories that fascinated me but could not be discussed at the dinner table. I also helped with infection prevention data, and prior to that I was trained as an Ebola Response Nurse in the ICU. Germs love me, and I love them. From a distance. In particular, I remember putting on the monkey suit to practice for an Ebola patient and laughing hysterically when the nurse manager brought out a roll of duct tape. "You're kidding, right?" I asked, incredulous.

"No, you put the duct tape around your wrists to get a good seal between the suit and your gloves. It's a really good seal that way," she explained, totally missing the humor of having your life depend on duct tape.

"Well, I guess it worked for NASA..." I joked. One of the things that amazes me about infections is the reinforcement of "clean" and "unclean" objects, just like the Bible discussed thousands of years ago. The instructions for dealing with mold in the Old Testament are nearly identical to the CDC instructions for managing mold after a hurricane has flooded one's home, except the ancient Israelites did not have bleach. Ancient Israelites were not supposed to touch anything dead, or they would be considered unclean; it took thousands of years to get European doctors to pause after studying a cadaver to wash their hands before heading over to deliver a newborn baby.

The most important rule of Biblical cleanliness was that pretty much no one could be clean enough to touch God, or even see Him. The Ark of the Covenant that carried His Presence inside could not be touched, or the person would immediately drop dead (1Chron. 13:10). The mountain where God came and gave the law to Moses could not be touched, or the Israelites would surely die (Ex. 19:12). The truth was that every human being was an untouchable.

Then came Jesus: He touched lepers and healed them yet followed the rules of authority by asking them to report to the priest for confirmation that they were truly clean. Then there was the woman with the issue of blood who said if she could only touch Jesus, she would be clean, but if this same woman had touched the Ark of the Covenant, she would have been struck dead. Yet, as Jesus walked by, the human dwelling place of the Presence of God, she touched Him, and she was healed—not struck dead. Jesus took someone untouchable and when He touched her, she became clean (Luke 8:44). I have never met a treatment that could work that quickly.

Those of us who work with germs have a lot of rules to remember. We must navigate antibiotic-resistance, sterilization procedures, reporting, and endless handwashing. Even as I scrub, brush, and cleanse, it can feel sometimes like trying to scrub away invisible sin. There is no amount of cleaning that could sterilize our sin, but God can deep-clean us to the spirit and marrow of our beings—and now He even lets us touch Him without dying. Before Jesus walked this planet, we were all equal in sin and death. Now, we are pulled up by the purity of His sacrifice on the cross to join a heavenly family of the redeemed.

Discussion Questions:

For Individuals or Groups

- Would you be afraid to touch Jesus? Why or why not?

- Have you asked God to purify you and forgive your sins? Take some time to pray about any sins that come to mind.

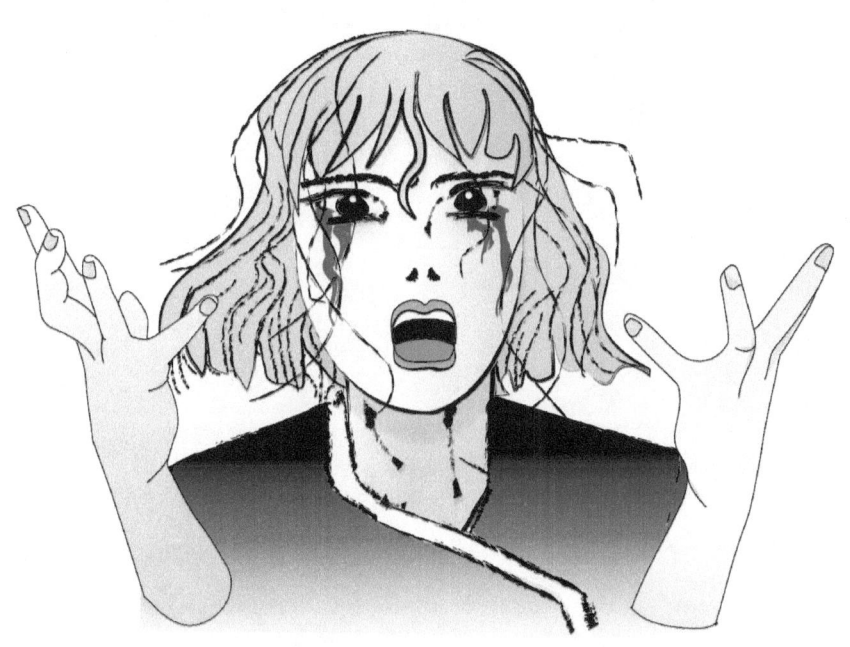

DARKNESS

These stories are about sin, fallen
people and spiritual darkness

One

SUSPICION

"By day the LORD commands his steadfast love, and at night his song is with me, a prayer to the God of my life." (Psalm 42:8) d by these you shall become unclean. Whoever touches their carcass shall be unclean until the evening." (Lev. 11:24)

At first, I thought it was a stomach bug or maybe just stress—my mother was in the hospital, and we were all worried about her. But instead of getting better, I found myself curled in bed in the fetal position, panting from the pain, and when I half-crawled to the bathroom to vomit, my father whisked me to the Emergency Department. It was actually my second trip because the first time I went to the ED the pain wasn't this bad, and they said it was probably just constipation and sent me home without testing. This time, I was sweating, nauseous, gray, and panting between moans.

I had never experienced such pain, and I had not been able to eat and keep it down in several days. When we settled in a room, the ED nurse told me with an irritated tone that I needed to control my breathing.

"I can't!" I said anxiously. "I don't know what's wrong."

"Yes, you can. You have control of your breathing, and you need to breathe slowly. You're hyperventilating, and that's why your hands feel numb." I nodded and tried to slow my breathing. Surprisingly, I found that she was right. I was just a teenager, and I felt out-of-control and desperate: Why was this happening to me? At least focused breathing gave me something to think about besides the pain in my belly. The nurse asked if I was sexually active, and I said "no." Then she sent my father out of the room and said I needed to be honest because my life might depend on it: Was I sexually active? "No," I shook my head adamantly.

"Listen, if you're not going to cooperate, it's going to be very difficult to care for you."

"I am being honest. Can my dad come back in now?" I felt scared because I was telling the truth. If honesty was important to my care, what would happen if they didn't believe me?

"Fine," she answered. "But we're going to run a pregnancy test on you, and we'll find out then anyway." Then she walked out of the room briskly, and I found myself alone and terrified. Soon, my father came in, and the doctor gave me the same grilling, telling me he was sure I had a pregnancy complication and that it would be "very helpful" if I would just be honest with them. They were frustrated and angry with me, but they glanced at my father every time it started to show. I felt they were assuming the worst of me, particularly because I was being completely honest. They thought I was keeping secrets when I had none.

The pain was still throbbing, and I couldn't find anyone in the ED who would believe what I was saying. It was utterly traumatizing to be an eighteen-year-old and have a doctor angrily conduct tests as though ready to shout, "ah-ha! We found you out, liar!" It turned out that I needed emergency surgery, and I was nearly septic—not a pregnancy complication. When they finally found out that I wasn't lying, the doctor looked stressed and a bit scared—a lot of time had been wasted in pursuit of an incorrect diagnosis. I don't remember much after that, but I remember waking up after surgery and being taken to the pediatric ward, which also felt odd—not that I wanted to be with the adults, but the children's toys and Hello Kitty scrubs made me feel infantile.

The pediatric nurse was really kind, though, and she offered me a movie selection while I devoured two sandwiches, three juice cups, and an applesauce. All the available movies were children's cartoons, so I selected The *Prince of Egypt*. In the movie, Moses's father-in-law explained that the tapestry of life looks messy on the back side, but when the tapestry is flipped over to see it from above, the pattern is revealed as a work of art. I bawled. It was a tough, lonely night of morphine withdrawal where I couldn't stop crying, but the message in the story of Exodus became a "song in the night" that helped me remember God's plan in spite of all my fear and confusion. I knew that these "plagues" I was suffering must somehow come together for a good purpose.

The next morning, the nurse said she had just found out that my mother was upstairs and asked if I would like to eat my breakfast with her. I was so grateful! They walked me to the second floor, and I sat with my mom eating hospital eggs and buttered toast in her room. I shared my salt packet with her because she was on a forced diet, and she shared her coffee with me because they didn't serve coffee in pediatrics. Then we sorted our IV poles and took a walk together down the hospital hallway while the nurses wondered what misfortune had brought us both to the hospital at the same time. On the other hand, we were both nearly ready to walk out of the hospital alive and well, so it could just as easily be seen as a blessing.

We discharged together and recovered fully, but I was shocked to find that many of my friends greeted me after this harrowing event with a compliment about how I looked "so healthy." I had vomited for a week and had emergency surgery—there was nothing healthy about it, but I had lost weight and that was apparently all that mattered? I looked gaunt and pale, and I determined that the rules of beauty were completely unreasonable when my most "healthy" appearance required a trip to the ED and the removal of an internal organ.

One of the most critical memories from that experience was the suspicion I experienced as a young, female patient, presumed to be lying. In nursing school, I learned that teen pregnancy really was the most common reason for a young woman's abdominal pain, so their assumption—while harsh in approach—was not invalid. Now, as I think about the difficulty of keeping so many secrets as a nurse, I realize that having to hold so much secrecy inside of me, and hearing so many lies, could easily make me callous and suspicious in the way I approach people. If I find myself assuming the worst of others before I have really had a chance to know them, I now recognize it as a sign of exhaustion. Confusion, rumors, and suspicion are not of God, for nothing is hidden from His sight (Heb. 4:13). Like Moses fleeing to Midian, sometimes I just need to get away and ask for some advice from people I love and respect and spend some time in prayer; I need to "flip the tapestry" and see God's perspective on things. Otherwise, I could easily treat my eighteen-year-old self with frustration and suspicion, potentially causing harm in the process. After all, if I break my back serving the sick but "have not love" (1Cor, 13:2), I could miss the point of my calling

Discussion Questions:

For Individuals or Groups

- Have you ever assumed the worst of a patient? Why? Was it a valid suspicion?

- Has someone assumed the worst about you? What did you learn from that experience?

Two

CONFRONTATION

"If possible, so far as it depends on you, live peaceably with all." (Rom. 12:18)

My preceptor at the nursing home calmly explained that the facility often did not carry the medications and feedings that were ordered for new residents admitting from the hospital. It was up to the nurse to order those resources before the weekend because it could be days before it came from an out-of-town supplier. I was told to "borrow" feedings from another patient if that should happen. Just the idea of taking feedings from someone else made me feel like a crummy thief, and I had no idea that finding basic resources would be such a challenge. Other times, I found myself covering every unit in the hospital to find things like IV poles when our census was full, and the units behaved like tribes owing favors to each other's chieftains whenever anyone came to borrow equipment. I had no idea who "owned" the equipment, I just knew that I had a full census and patients that needed equipment.

One of the hardest resources to find at the nursing home was narcotic pain medication; due to safety and tracking reasons the facility kept a low stock. This meant that when our patients converted to comfort measures over a weekend and needed regular doses of morphine, I often worried that we might run out because no deliveries would be coming in. Later, I understood the rationale for this low stock of narcotics, however.

Our new nursing director in the ICU was a young, edgy hipster who seemed to manage people surprisingly well despite his odd bursts of erratic energy. We were hopeful that we might get some stability after our last few directors were fired and escorted out by security in only a few months. One day, the new director walked into my patient's room when I was documenting at the desk. I immediately walked in to see if he had questions about my care—I assumed it was an audit of some sort. He said he was just "checking things out." I didn't leave because I felt like this was not typical, but another nurse called me to the desk to answer a physician phone call, and I had to leave the room. About two hours later, my patient ran out of sedation early—the tube was completely dry and at least 15 minutes too early. I had to write it up as an incident and notify pharmacy. The director left the hospital between two security guards two weeks later, fired for narcotic diversion; apparently, I was not the only nurse with stories of medications running dry early, and his presence in the room was the common thread. Eventually, he was caught syphoning off medications from the patients.

No one tells you when you go into nursing that some of your colleagues and managers will steal or harass to meet their agenda, but we had union nurses who stocked expired supplies during Joint Commission surveys just so they could pressure management, and management asked for dirt on nurses who spoke up about problems, just to discourage staff from speaking up. One moment, we were asked to "speak up" and the next, we were asked to not "stir up trouble." What confusion!

Sometimes I had to speak up about patient problems that the family or physician did not want to hear about. Sometimes I had to speak up about injustice, like a trend of women miscarrying while working on a specific unit. One time, the air conditioning at the hospital stopped working, and my unit was on the top floor of a now sweltering multi-story hospital. Fans were brought in, and we ran the ice machine continuously, trying to rush with makeshift ice packs to a completely full unit of fifty patients. I was the charge nurse that day, and I was still trying to get my mind around what was happening while our leadership team tried to make plans and determine the safest solutions.

Meanwhile, the summer heat combined with the whirring ventilators and other machines began to spew hot air all around us. It felt like a convection oven, and I feared for both the patients and employees trying to manage in the heat. It was also the weekend, and I was worried about how long it would take to fix the air conditioning. I continued to check in with my manager after taking report on the census and staffing. About two hours into the shift, I heard shouting from the back of the unit where the ventilation was worst. I ran back as a nurse aide came for a wheelchair. "Grace just went down," she rasped in the humidity. "She's conscious now, but she needs to be seen."

Grace was one of our best nurses, and I often asked her for advice. She was one of the nurses who "could just tell" what was going to happen to a patient by looking at them. I ducked into the room, and she was already dismissing us, "I'm fine, I'm fine. I just need to finish my med pass, and I'll sit and rest a bit and drink some more water." Her cheeks were flushed, she was breathing rapidly, clutching ice packs on her chest and sweating profusely. The hallway to the patients' rooms at this end of the ward was even hotter than the rooms themselves. I insisted that she be seen in the Emergency Department; she certainly wasn't going back to work. She gave in grudgingly (which was another sign she was in bad shape), and I wheeled her to the ED where she was treated right away. She looked up at me over a nebulizer and groaned, "I hope this doesn't cost me an arm and a leg. I'm so sorry to leave you short up there. Please take care of yourself and everyone else."

I assured her we would be fine. We divided her patients to avoid having any one person alone in the hottest wing, and the rest of the shift was better as nighttime brought cooler temperatures, and our patients finally got some rest. But I was livid. We were working in disaster conditions.

In the early hours of the morning, I started an email: I looked up the CEOs professional email address on the internal website and wrote a polite but assertive email asking for reassurance that Grace would not be billed for a single dime of tonight's ED visit since it was caused by the workplace environment. I wrote that the staff had worked very hard trying to keep patient temperatures down and sheets dry, despite tropical temperatures that left them thirsty and exhausted. I fully realized that I could be fired or blacklisted for sending an ornery letter directly to the CEO, but Grace didn't deserve a thousand-dollar bill for a work-in-duced health problem. I asked the secretary to read over my shoulder to make sure everything was accurate. She sucked in her breath when I hit send. "I hope I still get to work with you after this is done. I mean, you're not wrong—I just hope you don't get fired."

The next day, I received a very kind letter from the CEO thanking me for bringing the incident to her attention and letting me know that Grace had already been informed that the ED visit would not be billed. There was a contact listed for Human Resources in case Grace needed anything else. My manager also sent me a personal thank-you, saying that she appreciated it so much that I was looking out for the staff and to please continue to speak up about their needs. Wow, I was so grateful! The whole thing could have gone really poorly— my boss could have felt threatened by my complaint, the CEO may have sent me to Human Resources for disgruntled behavior—there were a thousand ways for everything to turn out poorly. I felt like my conscience would not let me rest if I did nothing, but I was surprised by kindness in return.

I was not always proud of the times I spoke up about my personal interests—sometimes those requests were ill-informed or just plain selfish. Other times, I just failed to be respectful, and it overshadowed a valid message. But I mostly have regrets about times when I didn't speak up and felt later like I maybe should have said something, said more, or tried harder. I have zero regrets about the times I spoke up for someone else's needs, though. In fact, some of my best memories as a nurse were times when I stood up tall to say something was wrong or that I thought someone could get hurt. I want to be willing to be a troublemaker when it could help the most vulnerable parties avoid trouble, and I think that kind of confrontation is exactly the kind we are supposed to willingly embrace.

Discussion Questions:

For Individuals or Groups

- Do you struggle more with keeping secrets, or with speaking up?

- What has been your experience when you have spoken up about the truth even when it was unpopular?

Three

NEAR MISS

"If I say, 'I will not mention him, or speak any more in his name,' there is in my heart as it were a burning fire shut up in my bones, and I am weary with holding it in, and I cannot." (Jer. 20:9)

I watched the worried wife care for her husband all night long after a car accident, but I knew that his young mistress was with him when the car crashed. The mistress visited during the day when the wife was working, and the wife spent all night caring for him after a long day at work. I was incensed that he would treat his wife that way, and she was so nice to him. I really wanted to tell his wife what he had done.

Discretion is a quality that God seems to value, yet no secret is hidden from God; I suppose discretion is just knowing when to talk and when to keep quiet. Remaining silent is a special struggle for nurses who are guardians of so much private information that even James Bond would buckle under the pressure of HIPAA regulations when everyone is clamoring for facts. There were days when I wanted to explode with some ugly truth, and there were other days when I wanted to drill my colleague for answers.

I often wondered how to walk that line as a Christian, and federal regulations didn't necessarily make it clear whether I should discuss the girlfriend in the car with the visiting wife. While visiting a retired battleship, I saw a poster from World War II hanging on the wall that read, "loose lips sink ships," meaning any conversation about the location or mission could get them all killed. I decided to keep quiet and focus on my job rather than start a soap opera in the ICU because I couldn't find any therapeutic reason to get involved. But it really bothered me, and I wondered if I made the right choice in keeping silent. It would have been easy to talk.

In contrast, one of the secrets we are supposed to tell is when we make a mistake, and self-reporting is the hardest kind of secret to tell. In the field of Patient Safety, there is a great deal of knowledge built by the reporting of a "near miss"—a moment where a mistake was caught and harm to a patient almost occurred. Those near misses help prevent harm from happening in the future and create a culture of learning from mistakes rather than placing blame on individuals. The benefit of being able to fix a repeatable problem for future patients comes from honest reporting of our errors, and anyone trained in reviewing adverse events knows how important it is to provide an open, non-punitive atmosphere where an honest interview can occur, and a plan of correction can be made together.

I enjoy learning new things and often volunteered to float to other departments despite the uncertainty that came with crossing over to an unknown way of doing things. When I floated, I didn't know the team dynamics, often could not find the printer, couldn't remember the phone extension for paging physicians, and always discovered too late that my PIN would not work on the medication dispenser without an extra call to the pharmacy.

One morning, I was especially excited to work with one of my favorite teams of nurses. Each of us had promised we would be working today as well, and we had made plans to order lunch together. I was looking forward to a great day with patients that I knew well, co-workers who would have my back, and a tasty lunch from a local restaurant. But the charge nurse put her arm around me with an apologetic smile and said, "It's your turn to float to the ED. They have four Progressive Care patients and an ICU patient holding over there. It's an overload, but I checked them, and they're quite stable. They just need us to help cover their drips until we get beds over here—but we can call you when lunch arrives," she added with a smile.

My shoulders slumped as I walked over to the ED, praying that God would help me. As with many facilities, relations between ED and ICU nurses were not superb at our hospital: We teased them mercilessly, and they ignored our requests. It didn't help relations that the area where they held ICU patients was ill-equipped and under-supplied even by ED standards. I knew it was going to be a tough day.

My report and handoff were delayed. I couldn't even find the nurse who had taken care of my patients. Apparently, she had already gone home after giving report to the charge nurse. The charge nurse was busy with an EMS report on a trauma patient, and she did not have a chance to give a report on who my patients were until more than an hour after the usual start time. She said she hadn't checked on them and didn't really know them, so all I really got in report was the bed number and diagnosis.

Medications were not available in the patient cubbies, there were no pitchers of water for patients to take their medications when their meds were available, and the printer wasn't working at all. I needed to print consents for a stat radiology procedure, do assessments, wean drips, and give meds. I was very, very behind before I even started.

I went into turbo mode. I was literally spinning on the unit to get everything done for my patients, trying desperately to prevent delays in their care. I was still overwhelmed when the charge nurse walked up with a smile and said she needed to give me more patients. I already had all five holding patients, and there were three ED nurses complimenting each other's nails at the desk. I told the charge nurse that she would need to call my supervisor to address the new patient assignment. She raised her eyebrows at me. I explained, "it is 11:30am, and I am just now delivering nine o'clock meds to Room 7."

"Oh," she smiled. "I didn't know you were busy!"

I took a deep breath, trying not to get angry. I was hungry, too, and wished I would be sitting down to a nice lunch soon, knowing very well that I would probably miss lunch altogether. "I don't want to cause delays with these patients, but I need to be safe. Once I pass these meds, I'm giving report, and I'll take a patient upstairs—then I can take another one in his place."

She nodded and called over her shoulder as she walked away, "Okay, well let me know if you need any help!"

I tried to focus, but it seemed that every time I tried to finish that 9 o'clock med pass, someone "more important" would interrupt me. The physician rounded. The radiology transporter was ready for my patient right now. The respiratory therapist needed a renewed order before my dyspneic BiPAP patient could receive their scheduled Albuterol. I finally made it to a quiet corner and closed the curtain to the patient's room, half-hiding at this point. I started scanning and dropping the meds into the medication cup as quickly as I could.

Suddenly, a shiver went down my spine like an electric shock. My hair stood on end. My feet tingled. Without thinking, I said, "Yes, Lord?" I looked down at the computer screen and saw a note in small type in the corner of the screen that said that the pill I was putting into my patient's cup should be cut in half before administering. I had completely missed it. It was a beta-blocker that would slow down the patient's heart rate and doubling the dose could have caused harm to my patient.

"Thank you, Lord," I whispered, tears of relief forming

in my eyes. I don't know how I instinctively knew that the electric feeling I had in my spine was God trying to get my attention, but I just knew. As I look back, I can see such clear protection from the Lord in many everyday matters like that medication pass. He protected my patient and my license that day, and He did it again and again through my career. He was always so faithful, even when I was being lousy: I certainly did not hear from Him because I was being righteous—I was having a bad day, and I had a crabby, cynical attitude. I had not actually asked for help (it was a matter of pride), and I felt bitter that no one sincerely offered help. I missed my team and had decided to stew about it rather than try to delegate.

It's actually a sign of burnout when I miss things that I normally would recognize, or nearly make a mistake: a "near-miss." It's a sign of inattention and loss of focus, but rather than fall into shame over my failures, I try to stop and recognize it as a God-given sign that I need rest. That time of rest might keep me from making a mistake that could cause permanent harm. There are definitely times when rest is impossible, but other times, I'm just trying to be tough, like that day in the ED, even though help was available. Now, I try to stop and drink some water, or get a bite to eat, and I remember that near-miss whenever my supervisor is asking if I can pick-up extra overtime shifts even though I know it might not be safe. I also try to plan some rest on my next day off so that I return to work with better focus.

One tactic for burnout is also a cause of burnout, depending on the situation: A lot of us make a change in our work environment, such as training in a new department or requesting transfer, just because the new environment and the need to learn new skills can help bring focus back into our work. But if change is too stressful, or when these tactics are not working, it is important to seek some help through a counselor or mentor.

The other support system that is vital for survival and burnout prevention is the local church; my church family has encouraged me, talked through my difficulties, and prayed for me when I was struggling. The Bible literally says, "Six days you shall labor, and do all your work, but the seventh day is a Sabbath to the LORD your God. On it you shall not do any work" (Ex. 20:9-10a). Ideally, we are created to focus and work hard all week then take a full day to hang out with our families, take naps, chat with friends, and skip doing the dishes. Going to church is a great way to recharge and find the support I need to continue serving the rest of the week, and it has pushed back the cloud of burnout many times in my nursing career.

Psalm 55:22 says, "Cast your burden on the LORD, and he will sustain you; he will never permit the righteous to be moved." It is so infinitely comforting to know that I can trust Him to be my righteousness, to stop me from causing harm, to protect me, and to watch over everything I do—even when I have stopped looking.

The charge nurse came back and announced that beds were ready for three of my patients. She took over getting them transferred out so that I could catch up on assessment documentation, and I was able to receive the remaining patients. I also reported the near-miss, and maybe that event improved care for future patients waiting for beds in the ED. Either way, I know that being honest about my mistakes helped me learn and become a better nurse, and I vowed that I would be quicker to recognize and state my needs in the future.

Discussion Questions:

For Individuals or Groups

- Read Psalm 55:22 again. When has God kept you from "being moved" or shaken by circumstances?

- Have you ever had to admit a mistake? What did you learn from the mistake or self-reporting experience?

Four

TERRIBLE SECRETS

"**B**ut what comes out of the mouth proceeds from the heart, and this defiles a person. For out of the heart come evil thoughts, murder, adultery, sexual immorality, theft, false witness, slander. These are what defile a person." (Mat. 15:18-20a)

One hot day on the medical floor, the ventilation system was whirring softly in the background as I started to assess my patient. He was malnourished and frail-appearing, and he had hardly spoken since he entered the hospital. My first task was to check his blood sugar and change the dressings on his fragile, dry skin. As I worked slowly and gently to peel the paper tape and unwind the gauze wrap on his arms, he started mumbling. I quickly found that as AIDS-related dementia set in, he was beginning to hallucinate and talk out loud. I tried to listen for any sign of pain as I worked to dress his wounds.

When I got report that night, my colleague told me about a list of doctors who had signed off or refused to see my patient because he had AIDS. In fact, he was dying of AIDS and had converted to comfort measures that day, but there were no family members or friends to call—he was completely alone. I frowned. Not only was I a Christian, but nurses don't pick or choose who we treat. If you're sick, you get a nurse. Period. I thought these doctors were petty for refusing to care for a dying man. What was the point of our profession if we did not take care of the sick and dying?

Nurses and doctors are highly respected in our culture. Once, a woman at church leaned in toward my two-year-old son and asked him, "Are you proud of your mama for being a nurse? She helps a lot of people."

He burst into dimples and announced with great confidence, "My mama sleeps at the hospital!"

Several families turned to stare disapprovingly at me. "Don't tell my manager," I half-whispered to the stunned woman. I later explained to her that I worked nightshift, and my son did not know exactly what I did; he was just proud of me for being his mom. My son didn't love me more because of my work—he loved picking me up in the morning, so I could clean up, eat breakfast, and start snuggling with him over a story. My husband also liked to make comments about working nightshift, calling me a "lady of the night" when he dropped me off for work. Just the same, when I entered the dark, empty halls of the hospital that night, I knew I would miss them both. I always did.

As I took care of my delirious patient in his private room, I found myself feeling very alone and missing my husband and son even more. My patient's diagnosis provided him with a spacious, albeit dark corner of the unit where we could store all of our isolation gear nearby. To get to this room, I walked down a long hallway, leaving the noise and bustle of the nurse's station, to the end of the hall where it became quiet, like entering a chapel. It felt hot in the room under a mask and an itchy, yellow isolation gown. I could feel my undershirt becoming damp with sweat. Beads of perspiration formed on my brow. I was trying to work quickly but carefully with the bulky gauze dressings, but his skin was prone to peeling unless I poured plenty of saline over the gauze first. These dressing changes were time-consuming and required lots of special care. I held his limp arm up as I worked to unwrap the old gauze and apply ointments.

I was reminded of other patients whose bandages I had changed: Changing dressings took time, and during that time I often enjoyed a pleasant bonding experience with my patients. I wished this man could speak coherently, so I could care for his soul as well as his body in these final hours. What life choices had brought him to this state? Could he forgive and find forgiveness before entering eternity? Suddenly, he began to mumble again. His eyes lit up, and he held up his arms on his own, forcing me to pause his dressing change. I looked up and was shocked to find a lecherous look on his face as he motioned with his one of his hands. He was calling to an imagined figure in the corner of the room. Confused, I leaned in to hear what he was saying. What was he asking for?

My breath caught and my heart pounded when I heard his words clearly. I started to cry under my mask. I felt short of breath as my eyes and nose filled, and a chilled feeling crept over my wet skin. My head was suddenly throbbing. The hair on my arms and neck stood on end. I felt like I needed to vomit. My patient was fantasizing about a young boy and telling him in a cooing voice how to please him. My patient was a pedophile. As he crooned and smiled, petting the air with his hands, I felt like that little boy was in the room with us, and his life was shattered as this toothless, sweaty man stole both his childhood and his future with greedy delight.

I quickly put tape on his last dressing and burst out of the quiet room just as he pulled his hand under the sheet and began to play with himself. I tried to take a deep breath and I could not. I was suffocating. I ripped the mask off my face; its red marks lingering on my wet face. I quickly and silently washed up and took my lunch break. I wanted to get off the unit and find someone to talk to. I clocked out and started walking down the long, dark, chemical-smelling hallways to the vending machines, hoping to see a friend. An acquaintance. Anyone. A distraction. Someone who would tell me everything was okay. Someone who would tell me that I didn't need to carry this burden.

As I was walking down the hall toward the breakroom, I was grateful to run into an old friend. She greeted me warmly and asked, "Say, are you taking care of the teenage kid in 112?"

"Maybe," I answered, distracted. I knew who she was talking about, and I had taken care of him the previous night.

"Yeah, well, my friend is his girlfriend, and she was wondering—what is he here for?"

I stared blankly.

Seeing my hesitation, she said, "Well, you know, she's worried."

I was so mad. In fact, I was furious. She knew that HIPAA meant we could not share information about patients. Why was she asking me to break the rules for something so trivial? Her question made me furious. There I was, sitting on a horrible secret about a patient that I was desperate to talk to someone about, and my friend wanted to know about a different patient just for gossip's sake. It was unfair; I had not done anything wrong. But I was angry at myself because I wanted to spill everything and resented my duty to keep quiet. Mostly, I was angry at that awful man for fantasizing about hurting children and possibly giving a terrible disease to them in the process. I felt a visceral disgust toward that miserable, dying man. And I didn't know if it was right to be silent about someone else's hell. I could just picture the boy he was talking to in the room, and he looked a lot like my beautiful son. What could I do? My face flushed again, and I wanted to run hard and not come back.

It felt horrible to stay silent, but I didn't know if it was right to talk either. My soul was screaming, and I just wanted to yell at this jerk who was taking advantage of her position as a secret-holder, breaking all the rules I was wrecking myself to keep, just to win favor with a friend. It would be so easy to talk because this kid, the teenager, was fine. He was going to go home tomorrow, and I couldn't even say that, much less unload about the pedophile upstairs. I was struggling with the long wait for justice, and I didn't know if I could hold on. I didn't know if I could just shrug and trust God on this one. I wasn't certain that I could have good character after tonight's shift.

I looked my friend in the eyes and tried not to cry. "You know I can't talk to you about that," I answered flatly. "She can call him herself and ask him how he's doing." She nodded, and I walked away briskly.

I finished my shift in near silence. When I went home, I cleaned up and held my son for a long time. I wished I could just stay home with him, protecting him from the evil world around us. I kissed his head and wished I could just be his mom and not listen to such terrible secrets.

I returned to work the next night to a man who had just died. AIDS had finally taken him. My colleague said he didn't speak at all the entire shift. I was just lucky, I guess. I cleaned his body and notified the authorities because he had no family or friends to contact. I called the funeral home that was working with the state, and they said he would be buried in a simple wooden box, and I shivered to think where his soul now resided.

I knew that I should've prayed for my patient that first night—before he died—but I just couldn't quite pray and mean it. I said the words, but my heart didn't really want him to be forgiven. I was angry at the evil in him, and just the thought of him repulsed me. In the end, death came to a sinful and unrepentant man, and I thought that it was just that God would give him what he deserved. Then God did something in me. A realization hit me hard: I was unable to pray for the soul of a dying man; I was just like the physicians who signed off and would not care for him. The doctors I had judged in the first five minutes of my shift were just like me; I was like them. I needed forgiveness.

From that point forward, whether or not I could pray for my patient became a litmus test for my attitude. If I found that I couldn't pray for a patient, I would ask the charge nurse if I could "take a minute" before taking over care of the patient. They never refused, and I used that minute to get my attitude right, praying about my heart and letting God take the bias and grudges off my back. Even then, sometimes, it takes more than a minute. Sometimes, it takes a lot longer.

To this day, I wonder if there was something I could have done, someone I could have called who could take those dirty secrets and deal out justice. But there really wasn't. Sometimes people compare nurses to priests because we hear people's deepest confessions. The difference is that when a nurse hears a confession, it is messy and angry and guilty. When beautiful repentance occurs, we usually call the chaplain to take over so the patient can find absolution with God. But HIPAA allows for no absolution. Nurses silently carry their patients' secrets, and if they do talk about a patient, the details must be changed, redacted, and depersonalized into parable-like case studies like this one, to protect patient identities. But despite washing the information of all the personal details, the secrets linger.

When I had a patient who had an especially odorous GI bleed, another senior nurse explained how to deal with lingering bad smells. We wanted to hold ourselves together without making rude noises while changing this poor patient: After washing thoroughly, we applied a small amount of menthol rub on the skin just beneath our nostrils and then applied a face mask as a barrier. With this technique, we were not overwhelmed by the smell, and we cheerfully changed the patient's linens. In a lot of ways, terrible secrets are like bad smells—the best way to handle them is to apply something good and focus on it, applying a soft barrier as needed. This need for goodness is why I memorized this scripture from Philippians:

> "Finally, brothers, whatever is true, whatever is honorable, whatever is just, whatever is pure, whatever is lovely, whatever is commendable, if there is any excellence, if there is anything worthy of praise, think about these things." (Phil. 4:8)

I have heard many terrible things as a nurse, but I have witnessed indescribable love and beauty as well. I have watched saints pass from earth into heaven, miraculous recoveries, and profound strength and endurance through extreme difficulties. Now I focus on the good and remember the people who astounded me for their character and legacy, and it helps a great deal.

Before I had to keep secrets, I had always wondered about this one passage in Revelation where all of heaven starts weeping. Why would there be weeping in heaven? They wept because they could not find anyone worthy to open the scroll of judgment. This was the scroll that would tell all the secrets—but no one could bear it. No one was worthy. Then suddenly, the Lamb appears, stained with blood and completely pure. Heaven erupts in celebration as he takes the scroll,

> "And they sang a new song, saying, 'Worthy are you to take the scroll and to open its seals, for you were slain, and by your blood you ransomed people for God from every tribe and language and people and nation." (Rev. 5:9)

In the Lamb of God, they did not only find purity, authority, and judgment, but stunning redemption as well. He stepped down from heaven and died for us on earth. One day, God will reveal every secret as His Son—the only One who is worthy—judges the world, so that everything that was hidden in the dark is shown in the light. He is not only just, but merciful.

It's satisfying to know that truth and justice will come. It's comforting to know that it will be both fair and merciful. But I really believe the hardest part is the lack of closure. Were my prayers answered? Will I see my worst patients in heaven, forgiven, with changed hearts? Will the ones who were harmed by evil men be comforted? True comfort can only come from the hands of the Lamb who is worthy, and having my eyes opened to real suffering from sin as a nurse has placed a real longing in my heart for a day when God will comfort His broken creation:

> "He will wipe away every tear from their eyes, and death

shall be no more, neither shall there be mourning, nor crying, nor pain anymore, for the former things have passed away." (Rev. 21:4)

"The Spirit and the Bride say, 'Come.' And let the one who hears say, 'Come.' And let the one who is thirsty come; let the one who desires take the water of life without price." (Rev. 22:17)

Discussion Questions:

For Individuals or Groups

- Read Revelation 5:9. Why is all of heaven relieved when the Lamb of God appears? What does it mean when they say, "He alone is worthy? "

- Read Exodus 34:6-7 where God passes by Moses. Can you imagine if God was only compassionate and not just, or if He was only just and never merciful? What would heaven be like without both?

Five

CONFRONTING EVIL

"**I**f we say we have fellowship with him while we walk in darkness, we lie and do not practice the truth. But if we walk in the light, as he is in the light, we have fellowship with one another, and the blood of Jesus his Son cleanses us from all sin." (1John 1:6-7)

I walked into my patient's room to check their vitals and adjust their drips, but I nearly stumbled over a pile of coals placed prominently just under the foot of the hospital bed. The entire family sitting around the patient jumped to their feet in alarm. I sighed, resisting the urge to kick them across the floor: They looked like giant, black bugs. Instead, I gingerly scooted them further underneath the bed to prevent falls. Apparently, the witch doctor had placed them there to remove the curse that was afflicting my patient's health. It was just another day caring for people in a superstitious society. I had seen a lot over the years. Eggs were used in divination to find out the gender of a baby in the womb. If someone's high-heeled shoes snapped, my co-workers would shake their heads sadly because they knew someone had given that poor woman the evil eye. Most hospitals have a place that employees swear is haunted, usually by a Catholic nun. Some of my patients swore that a nun appeared to them and then disappeared in the night. The local animal shelter refused to permit the adoption of black cats until after Halloween because a death cult might use them in ritual sacrifices over the holiday. I was told that a few years ago, several young people had been kidnapped for the same purpose; a claim I sincerely doubted until I looked it up and found it to be true. Terrifying.

Despite these ghost stories, the Bible is quite clear that Christians should never practice witchcraft, drink blood, or seek answers from a medium (Lev. 19:26, 31). Saul knew the rules when he went straight to the witch of Endor for answers when God was silent (1Sam. 28:7). God had already delivered a message of judgment to Saul, but he desperately wanted a better outcome. A wise preacher once said that when God is silent, we had better make sure that we have obeyed the last thing God told us to do because He is not obligated to repeat Himself. When the hospital is oppressive and evil surrounds us, the last thing we want to do is silence our faith and stop listening to God, so it is important to live obediently in His will, turning away from anything that would pull us down when we need to face the darkness (Heb. 12:1).

In the shadows of evening, when nurses sit down to a quiet, candle-lit dinner together, we have a lot of strange experiences to sort through. We have questions. We often share our most unsettling stories in whispers with each other because we can hardly speak about them with others. On one such night, a few of us were gathered for dinner around a single candle surrounded by empty dessert plates, and we leaned over our coffee cups to listen:

"The man was born blind, so of course he had never seen anything at all." A tall man with glasses was speaking about his days in the operating room. "He coded on the table, but we brought him back almost immediately. Imagine our surprise when the recovery nurse called us because we 'really needed to hear this.' Well, that blind man described coming out of his body, floating up, and seeing—seeing!—everything around him. He recited the credentials on our name tags and what color the curtains were, and all kinds of details about the operating room where he had been sedated. Then he found himself suddenly rushing back into his body and was blind again! We had no explanation: When he was dead, he could see." The tall man took a sip of coffee, shaking his head in disbelief, signaling that his story was finished.

Another nurse cleared her throat, "One time, my colleague came running out of the room screaming, 'That man is possessed! He's talking in English!' We laughed because we had no clue what she was talking about, but apparently, the man was very poor, spoke only Spanish, and could not read or write. While she was preparing medication in the room with him, he started speaking in a high voice, and it sounded like French. She was really confused and stopped what she was doing to check him. Then he turned and looked right at her and spoke in a different, deeper voice in perfect English. Well, she ran right out of the room, and you know the rest." She shrugged with a smile, "I never knew what he said to her that made her so scared."

"Oh, I remember running out of the room for help once because my patient kept screaming for help and would not stay in bed. He said that the devil had come to take him and begged us to help him. I went to the door and called for help to hold him down, but just then he coded and died. Do you think that's really what happened?" We stared silently at the candle on the table and shivered. How could we know such things?

Instead of answering, I shared my own story: "I was interrupted from my lunch break when we admitted a tiny woman that no one could restrain," I began. "My coworker had just been telling me about her dating life, trying to find a good Christian man to marry, and how she secretly worried that she would never marry or have children. When the charge nurse called for help, we dropped our lunches and quickly ran to the room to find a tiny, frail woman writhing in the bed, jerking the other nurses around like ragdolls. She was extremely strong, and we had to call the house supervisor because she had broken the cloth restraints. Her medications were not doing anything to calm her down. She was moaning in a small, high voice. We couldn't imagine how such a tiny woman could be so strong! As we carefully applied leather restraints so that we could safely assess her and administer medications, she turned her head and looked directly at my friend. She spoke in a deep, man's voice and said, 'You are cursed! You will never have children, and no one will ever love you!' My friend cried out and ran from the room in tears as the patient collapsed in the bed, suddenly weak and tired, no longer straining against us. Later, I joined my friend, and we prayed and worshipped together because God is bigger than our enemies, even the ones we do not understand."

"I'm glad you did that," a young woman nodded. "I have found that singing praise songs can calm a lot of the wildness in those sorts of patients."

"Just like David and Saul," I added.

We all nodded in agreement. "And sometimes it takes more than just prayer to get through the shift," the tall man added.

All of us sitting around the table that night were taught that the hospital was a place of science where there was no room for superstition or religion. But spiritual realities were all around us, many of them quite dark—even evil. Without my faith, I would have felt lost. I didn't understand why people around us were inviting witch doctors to cast spells, but Christians were forbidden to even mention prayer; it sounded a lot like Daniel's time when jealous leaders convinced King Darius to make a rule banning prayer to anyone but the king, just so they could trap Daniel (Dan. 6:7-8). Yet, Daniel continued to pray to God (v. 10); he feared the Lord more than lions.

Somehow, many of us started to fear the lions of hospital administration and the state nursing board more than God.

We believed that we need to ask permission to practice our faith and walk with Him. But as Christians working in a hospital surrounded by life and death all day long, why would we give up the one weapon we have and succumb to the darkness? Why would we take off our armor before battle (Eph. 6)? The last thing I wanted to do when I walked in the valley of the shadow of death was to hide in the shadows.

The Bible says that there really is a lion lingering in those shadows:

"Your adversary the devil prowls around like a roaring lion, seeking someone to devour. Resist him, firm in your faith, knowing that the same kinds of suffering are being experienced by your brotherhood throughout the world." (1Pet. 5:8b-9)

The lion we must face comes "to steal and kill and destroy" (John 10:10), and that reality can be awfully dark, but just like Daniel in the lion's den, we are not alone. Remember the words of David, "Even though I walk through the Valley of the Shadow of Death, I will fear no evil, for you are with me" (Psalm 23:4). Believers throughout time and around the world experience the same struggles. The spiritual world is real, and we cannot restrain it with cloth or sedatives or laws or even scientific reasoning. But at the sound of His Name, the demons flee, giants fall, and lions are kept at bay. The battle belongs to the Lord.

And why does God put us into this battlefield in the first place? What happens to the ones that face this darkness without Him? My Christian co-worker was able to pray, worship, and recover; a demonic curse became a misfired enemy bullet. But someone else, without Christ, may have been seriously injured. With Christ, it is important to be aware of the enemy in the shadows hoping to kill us, but we do not need to be afraid, for our God walks beside us carrying His rod and His staff. One day, the kingdom of the world will become the kingdom of our Lord (Rev. 11:15), and we will dwell in His house forever (Psa. 23:6).

Discussion Questions:

For Individuals or Groups

- What spiritually unsettling stories do you know?

- Read Hebrews 12:1: Is there any sin clinging to you that needs to be cast off so you can run freely?

- Do you need to repent for any spiritually dark activities (mediums, witchcraft, etc.)? Have you removed them from your life?

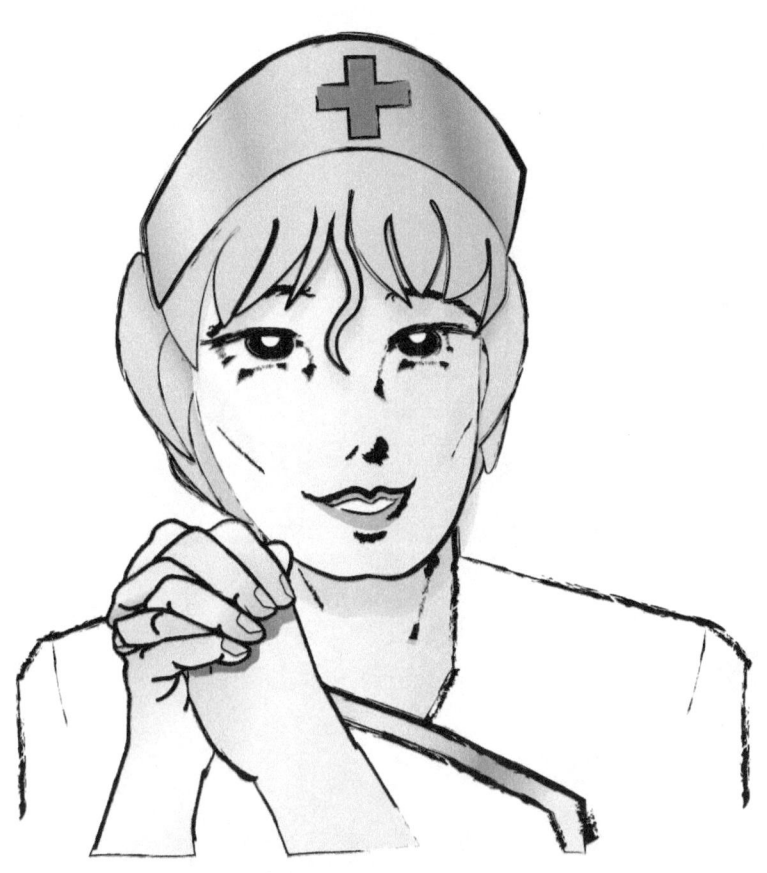

DISCHARGE

These stories are on the topic of
preparing for eternity

One

WEDDING CLOTHES

"But when the king came in to look at the guests, he saw there a man who had no wedding clothes. And he said to him, 'Friend, how did you get in here without a wedding garment?' And he was speechless." (Mat. 22:11-12)

I stood in line to checkout at Wal-Mart on a very busy day with crowds of people all around. I was tasked with picking up some last-minute items for an office birthday party, and I was trying to hurry, but the long lines held me back. I took a deep breath, stood with my feet apart in a comfortable stance, and prepared to wait awhile.

Suddenly, someone hollered and waved to me. "I can check you out over here!"

I looked around and pointed at myself. "Me?"

"Yes, of course! I can check you out right here," she

answered cheerfully.

I walked cautiously past the crowd of customers into a newly opened checkout lane and purchased my few items. I smiled and said thank you very much. "Bye! We'll see you soon!" the employee called after me. I arrived at work in good time and wondered all day about the expedited checkout—where did this unexpected favor come from? Why was the employee smiling during one of the busiest times of the day? Why me?

After several cups of coffee, I suddenly needed to speed-walk to the ladies' room. It was a short walk through artificially-lit hallways with abstract art to reach the restroom in the hospital's administrative wing. As I walked into the restroom, I glanced at the wall-to-wall mirror and stopped. Staring back at me with an open mouth and a silly grin was a woman dressed in button-up navy-blue blouse over tan pants. I giggled nervously—I was dressed like a Wal-Mart employee! The morning's events came flooding back. It was as if I had unintentionally gone undercover at the big box store to obtain a handful of trinkets in rapid time. I was a secret shopper—a spy of sorts, undercover as a Wal-Mart native. How clever and idiotic!

One of my mentors used to tell me that half of life is about showing up on time, and the other half is about being dressed for the job. Her experience only highlighted my inability to notice such details in my wardrobe. My fashion sense is infamously lacking. In a famous parable, Jesus tells the story of a king who hosts a wedding banquet for his son: He sends his servants to tell those who were invited, "I have prepared my dinner ... everything is ready. Come" (Mt 22:4). But they paid no attention and were punished for their disrespect. Then the king invited anyone from the streets, bad and good, and the banquet was filled with guests. But the king noticed a poor man who was not wearing wedding clothes and questioned him. The man couldn't think of any excuses, and he was promptly thrown out of the banquet "into the outer darkness. In that place there will be weeping and gnashing of teeth. For many are called, but few are chosen" (Mat. 22:13b-14).

I identify with the shabby folks who are scared of the king's men but fascinated by an invitation to hob-nob with the royal family. I can also say that the wedding of Christ and the church is a time when I do not want to make a fashion faux pas. I look to Revelation 7:14 to get a hint on heavenly etiquette: "These are the ones coming out of the great tribulation. They have washed their robes and made them white in the blood of the Lamb." In opposition to this image, another passage in Isaiah 64:6 declares, "all our righteous deeds are like a polluted garment" (the ancient term for soiled menstrual cloths). Personally, I would rather wear a white robe to the party than soiled feminine pads!

Thank God we can accept the invitation to the banquet even though we are shabby, but we are required to accept his new clothes and have our sins washed in the holiness of Jesus's blood; the Bible warns us not to show up at the party without the righteousness of Christ. I hope I never accidentally wear the competitor's uniform in the checkout line, and I want to check my spiritual closet to make sure I am ready for the ultimate party.

Discussion Questions:

- Have you ever failed to dress properly for an event? What happened?

- Have you asked Jesus to forgive your sins and make you ready for heaven?

Two

THE BEACH

"My sheep hear my voice, and I know them, and they follow me. I give them eternal life, and they will never perish, and no one will snatch them out of my hand." (John 10:27-28)

My 5-year-old son clasped my hand tightly and looked jealously at his one-year-old sister, who was sitting on my hip, a comfortable distance from the hot sand.

"Go—Run and play!" I encouraged him.

He shook his head violently. "It's scary."

Before us, gentle ocean waves sparkled and lapped at the giant beach where families could be seen running into and out of the surf, laughing, and resting in the sunshine. The waves made a soft but giant roar that dwarfed their words. Looking out, the water seemed to stretch out forever into a distance never seen by this small family. We stood, watching, and as we looked out at the ocean, the swimsuit-clad laughter faded and all that we could see was vastness. As my son began trying to climb my leg like a tree, I prayed for a way to comfort him.

I looked down into the eyes of my son, blue-green like the ocean, they were wide and filled with terror. It was all just so big, and he was still so small. His face was pleading with me to get back into the safety of the car. "Hey! Do you know what?" I asked enthusiastically.

"What, Mama?" he asked undeterred, continuing to climb.

"Do you know what I think when I see this giant, scary ocean, and I see how big it is, and how small I am?"

"What?" he paused a moment to listen.

"I think…Wow! God made this!" I spread my hand out before the view. "He said a word, and a GIANT ocean and a beach and all this sky was made. Can you even imagine a God that's so big he can make oceans just by talking?" My son shook his head, standing still and listening intently now. I leaned close and whispered, "and when I think of how huge God is, there is one more thing that I think of next."

"What is it?" he whispered back.

"That same God that is so big that He can just say a word and make an ocean is the God who loves you and me with the biggest, strongest love we can ever imagine."

I paused to let that sink in.

"Isn't God amazing?" I spoke softly to my son, who was

now quiet as I put a hand on his tousled head.

"He is! He's huge and awesome and scary, and he LOVES me!" My little boy instantly leaped off of me and threw his arms in the air, twirling on the sand.

"Awesome!" I returned, smiling at his dancing.

"Wow! God is big! Woo-hoo!" My son hollered at the top of his lungs, absolutely giddy with joy. We held hands and ran into the waves, skipping into and out of the lapping current. My baby girl began to giggle a deep, guttural laugh as we bounced in the spray.

Sometimes, when someone is dying, it's like looking out at a giant ocean, and you can't tell what's below the surface of the water. There's no warning when the weather turns, and dark clouds sweep over ominously. It is terrifying unless you know the One who made the storm clouds and all the giant fish hidden beneath those turbulent waves. God made all of this, and it's okay that we don't understand it all. He is big, I am small, and that's okay because He loves me. My eyes search the horizon for the shore to come and focus on the face I long to see most: Jesus.

Discussion Questions:

For Individuals or Groups

- What is the biggest thing you have seen in this world? The ocean? Grand Canyon? The night sky? A forest? Did it scare you?

- Praise God for making such grand creations and still loving us though we are small.

Three

DISCHARGE DISPOSITION

"We all fade like a leaf, and our iniquities, like the wind, take us away." (Isa. 646b)

The smells of aerosolized medication filled the air with a steamy odor. The light over the sink was on, leaving most of the room in shadows as the BiPAP pumped, hot and even like a heartbeat. It was about two o'clock in the morning, and I was the charge nurse for the nightshift. The primary nurse, Serenity, was trying to coach her hypoxic COPD patient to take slow, deep breaths, so the medication would work better, but he was very anxious. His behavior and insomnia were expected because he was on hospice for his condition—but oxygen, Ativan, Morphine, and a respiratory treatment were still not helping him calm down. He was strong enough to sit up in a chair, and we were hoping to help him rest a bit that night. Truthfully, he was not just anxious, but very angry. I have seen anger and paranoia in hypoxic patients before, though, and we took it in stride: It wasn't personal—it was just a manifestation of his physical ailments. But I could tell that Serenity would definitely need some help tonight because this patient was quite strong and looked like he might strike out at us if things escalated.

We talked patiently to him about positioning for comfort, medications we were giving, checking his vitals, and counting his breaths together. He gave curt nods, clearly exasperated with the instructions but still working with us, and we were determined to stay and work with him as long as he needed. About fifteen minutes later, he tore off his BiPAP mask, and suddenly threw it at Serenity, shouting at us: "I'm ready to die. Just F***ing stop it and let me die!"

We backed off and let him talk, carefully reaching for the mask to keep it from dropping on the floor and becoming dirty. He took a slow, wheezy breath, and suddenly expletives were spilling out of his reddened face in a choppy, violent rush. Then he cursed God at the top of his lungs, shaking his fist, until he slumped over in the chair. Serenity and I both rushed to him and checked his pulse and pupils: He was dead. His last words were riddled with profanity, anger, and violent fury. Serenity and I just looked at each other, horrified in the eerie silence, waiting for some sort of resolution. As a Do Not Resuscitate (DNR) hospice patient, there was nothing more to do.

Eventually, we moved his body to the bed for postmortem care and completed the required paperwork and notifications.

His son was irritated when we woke him up with a phone call to notify him of his father's death. Shaken, Serenity and I went through the motions as though nothing had happened, but we were both pale and quiet for the rest of the shift. I wondered if God would judge this patient to be "not in his right mind" when he died, or if I had just witnessed a man going into eternal judgment in hell.

One of my nursing professors taught me to ask the question, "What is keeping this patient from going home?" every day, for every patient. Keeping the goal of discharge in mind is a unique perspective that immediately prioritizes the otherwise lengthy list of patient problems and interventions. In healthcare, this emphasis on patient outcomes is based on the fact that all patients either discharge or die, and nearly every patient who enters the hospital hopes to leave the hospital alive. It's the same in life, because there are only two destinations for our souls, heaven or hell, and everyone wants to go to heaven. I never like to think about the second option, and I try to avoid talking about it, but every human being will discharge to one of these eternal homes. What barriers do they face before discharge from earth? This perspective definitely prioritizes all my problems to put eternity into focus as the final goal.

But when that patient died cursing God, I felt a little bit of the horror that Jesus reveals in the parable of the rich man and Lazarus, where the rich man dies and goes to hell (Luke 16:19-31). He begs Abraham to send Lazarus with a bit of cold water because he is "in anguish in this flame" (v. 24). Abraham explains that it is not possible for Lazarus to cross over the chasm between heaven and hell, so the rich man asks Abraham to warn his brothers. Abraham says that Moses and the prophets have already warned his brothers and further warning is not needed. But the rich man begs once more to let someone go to warn his brothers from the realm of the dead because his brothers will surely repent if someone comes back from the dead to warn them. I think it is such beautiful mercy that Jesus raises a man named Lazarus from the dead, almost as if it is a response to the rich man's request (John 11:44).

In a similar illustration, one of the criminals crucified next to Jesus acknowledges his guilt, and Jesus tells him, "Today you will be with me in Paradise" (Luke 23:43). But the criminal on His other side is a different story: He rails against Jesus, telling Him to "Save yourself and us," implying that Jesus is just another criminal and probably a liar (Luke 23:39). I don't like to read that passage—I like to skim right down to the promise of paradise. But two men hung next to Jesus and both men faced their final judgment that night. I think this reality, combined with my own experience with death and wanting to know that I was ready, is why I feel so strongly about listening for opportunities to talk with people about their souls before it's too late.

Patients in hospitals today are nearly an unreached people group; as a patient, I found that it was extremely difficult to find anyone in the hospital who would engage in a conversation about my spiritual concerns. Many professionals fear they will say something wrong, so they do not speak at all. But I also learned that there are a lot of Christians working in hospitals who look for opportunities to help, to offer chaplain services, to pray with patients, and to talk with them about whether there is anything they want to do to prepare for the possibility of chronic problems, or even death. Patient outcomes matter, and the most important outcome is the one that lasts for eternity.

Discussion Questions:

For Individuals or Groups

- Do you think the story of the patient who cursed God before he died was purely a physical manifestation, or a spiritual one as well? Why or why not?

- Do you think patients are an "unreached people group"?

Four

FROZEN BRANCHES

"I am the vine; you are the branches. Whoever abides in me and I in him, he it is that bears much fruit, for apart from me you can do nothing." (John 15:5)

Recently, there was a terrible freeze in our area that left many without power and decimated fields, orchards, and gardens. As we cleaned up, we asked friends and neighbors what to do with the dead Hibiscus plants in our front yard because I am clueless about gardening. They explained that if we cut down the dead branches, the larger branches may have signs of life and recover fully. They explained how to cut back the bark until we found living branches and to trim to that point and water them well. Then they warned us that if we left the dead branches on the plant, it would not recover, because the plant would put nutrients and energy into those dead branches and the living branches would die.

You don't feed a dead branch; you cut it off to save the living. Wow.

This has such a profound parallel to casting off sin and everything that weighs down the soul to focus all our energy into God's glory. I have heard that monkeys are extremely difficult to catch, but if someone leaves a banana in a cage with narrow bars, they will flatten their hand and reach in to grab the fruit. But because their closed hand is too large, they will not be able to pull it out without dropping the banana. They will hold onto the fruit and not let go; they will let themselves be captured, though they are not caged, because they will not let go of that banana. I had a patient with a similar approach to sin. He dove head-first through a deputy's rear car window, breaking through and escaping, only to have a seizure from the head injury—he was only a few feet away from the car, but he was willing to risk everything to avoid being caught by the authorities and go back to his life of drugs and crime. Others were treated for septic shock at their drug injection sites, only to rip their IVs out as soon as they could walk again—not even finishing their antibiotics, so they could go back to the streets and obtain drugs.

The reality is that the drug-seekers were the hardest patients for most of us. Every nurse would rather take care of a GI Bleed, a woman screaming in labor, or even a strong man with aggressive delirium than a drug-seeker. It cuts your heart open every time they beg for the next high. You can never tell if they are in physical pain—and they clearly are in pain from addiction, withdrawal, and spiritual hurt—or if you will harm them trying to provide comfort through medication. To see someone put every ounce of energy to dance closer and closer to death is enough to really burn-out a caring person.

One patient had a friend sneak drugs into the hospital, only for the patient to have a bad trip. He screamed all night long about bugs crawling on him and terrified the other patients on the unit. Another woman tried smoking pot in the bathroom with her oxygen tank tucked in with her. Another patient started cursing, threatening, and removing her clothes at the nurse's station to make us give her sedatives. One mixed her opioid tablet in water and injected it from a syringe in the trash, dying instantly from the embolus. Many patients would cry or yell, ordering the nurse to "push it fast," and instructing the nurse that they planned to be in pain again in four hours and to just bring the medicine even if they were calmly sleeping.

A patient that I will never forget was a twenty-something young man who had a stroke from using stimulants. He had a permanent expression of horror on his face, and his body was contracted and could barely be moved. Another man came to the hospital with headaches, only to find that his nasal passage had rotted away from snorting cocaine—it had formed a cavity that went straight into his brain, and he had to have a flap surgically placed to protect his brain, with IV antibiotics to treat the self-inflicted meningitis. Self-harm is so much more difficult to witness because the story could be so different. No one is born that way, but it forms over a series of choices—a desire to perform better in school, feel belonging, forget some past trauma, or to just feel good—all contained in a person who has a God-given purpose and an eternal soul.

My great-grandfather was an alcoholic. When he drove his kids into town to pick up Christmas dinner and buy presents, he told them to wait outside in the middle of bitterly cold winter weather. He went into the bar and did not come out until morning, all the money spent. Later, my grandfather had to cut his father down in the barn when he attempted to hang himself. The whole family was starving and hopeless. But one night, my great-grandmother took the kids to a tent meeting to hear a concert and a guest speaker. They lived in the country and any event of this magnitude was worth attending—even if it was religious. Toward the end of the evening, while the preacher was still speaking, my great-grandfather appeared in the back of the tent.

I often imagined him disheveled, unshaven, and smelling of alcohol, standing there amidst a crowd of people in their finest church clothes. He was weeping. The whole family watched as their alcoholic husband and father nearly ran to the front, telling the preacher that he wanted to be saved— that he knew he was a sinner, and that he needed God to save him. My great-grandfather was never the same. He became a full-time preacher after that, traveling with his family to sing and preach every day of the week. They stood in the streets and preached, they sang in tents, and traveled far and wide to share the message that God can save anyone, even a hopeless drunk.

He never drank another drop of alcohol after that day. He was illiterate and could not read the newspaper, but after that day he was miraculously able to read the Bible. My grandfather followed in his steps, and by the time I was born, our family was full of blessings: We enjoyed good marriages, plenty of food, education, and daily thanksgiving to the God who gave His Son's blood in exchange for a sinful man's soul.

If you are struggling with addiction today, I want to encourage you. We do not judge you. We cry and pray for your soul because we can see what God sees—you were made for more. God has a purpose for you and the power to heal. In Revelation chapter one, John sees the glorified, glowing, white-robed Jesus and falls at his feet. Jesus says "Fear not, I am the first and the last, and the living one. I died, and behold I am alive forevermore, and I have the keys of Death and Hades" (Rev. 1: 17b-18). God holds the keys to your hell, and he can unlock your soul and set you free forever. He knows what it is to be dead, He knows what it is to conquer death and hell, and He knows what it is to really live. He is First and Last, and He has seen it all—nothing you are or have done is shocking to him, and no sin is too big for him to heal and forgive. I tell you today, cut off the dead branches of addiction and put your life in the hands of Jesus. He has the power to unlock your soul and set you free.

This truth is why I became a nurse in the first place. I never had what it takes—I am far too sensitive, and I found myself weak and fearful in real life. But God told me to become a nurse, and I trusted His purpose for my life. At the end of my life, I want Him to tell me that I was a good and faithful servant (Mat. 25:23), and I figured I would have to be willing to risk failure and suffering to be in that group. I was fortunate to have a family history of failures who gave up their lives for God's glory as an example. Who can make a preacher out of an alcoholic? God can. Who could take an anxious hypochondriac and make her a nurse? God can. He cut off my frozen, dead branches and saved my life, and He can do the same for you.

Discussion Questions:

For Individuals or Groups

- Do you know someone who struggles with addiction? How can you pray for them today?

- What "dead branches" or failures are there in your life? What would it look like to prune them?

Five

INHERITANCE

"Do not lay up for yourselves treasures on earth, where moth and rust destroy and where thieves break in and steal, but lay up for yourselves treasures in heaven, where neither moth nor rust destroys and where thieves do not break in and steal. For where your treasure is, there your heart will be also." (Mat. 6:19-21)

When I think about this verse and storing up treasures in heaven for our heavenly reward, I often think of something that a persecuted Christian from the underground church said about evangelism. He said that bringing the message of salvation to others was part of our heavenly inheritance; if he did not obey the call to share, his inheritance in heaven would be so small. I confess that I do not know how such things work in heaven, but the thought intrigues me because I had a similar dream about heavenly rewards when I was a child. In the dream, I was with friends and family, and we were taking a walk in a beautiful golden field. I love to take walks, and we were picking the plants, casually harvesting as we went. It was a beautiful day. Eventually we noticed that on the other end of the field, there was a huge machine driving along and plowing down the plants. We started hurrying to pick what we could before the huge plowing machine got closer. The closer we came to meeting that machine, the faster we went, until we started running through the field, grabbing what we could harvest before we collided. I awoke just before we met the destructive machine. I prayed about the meaning of the dream and realized that if God has placed the souls of people on my heart, surely it's time to start running. I am meant to feel urgent about this harvest. I might not reach everyone I pass, but if I start running now, I may reach one more before the end.

There are times when I meet a patient, and I just know that they need to talk. Usually, they ask if they are going to die. I say something like, "When you find yourself in the hospital, it's a reminder that everyone dies at some point. I don't know if this is your time or not, but if it was, is there anything you would want to do before that happens? Is there anyone you want to call or forgive? Think about it, and if there is anything you want to take care of, I will help you, okay?" Believe it or not, my patients were not so anxious or scared after those conversations. They already knew what I said was true. In fact, they seemed to feel more calm about their hospitalization after discussing their questions. Sometimes I think the biggest stressor on our bodies is when our souls are in turmoil; it is a physical relief to address those concerns, and patients want to discuss it and find peace.

Most of my patients walked out of the hospital and went home to their families, but they all had this precious moment in the hospital to consider their mortal lives. They had a chance to stop and think about whether they wanted to change anything about their lives before they faced eternity or discharged home. A lot of patients frustrate their physicians by saying that people only go to hospital to die, but truthfully, anyone who goes to the hospital is walking in the shadow of death. As nurses, we work in the shadow of death everyday. But we can walk in the shadow of death and fear no evil, for He is with us (Psalm 23:4).

I was riveted by the story of Dr. Kent Brantly, a young doctor who stayed in Africa during an Ebola epidemic to work day-and-night with the sickest patients in harsh conditions. A documentary about the epidemic, Facing Darkness (2014), described Franklin Graham's commitment to the African people: As Christians, "we run to the fire; we don't run away from it." Dr. Brantly and his colleagues believed that God could be glorified in their service, and that they should not fear. Dr. Brantly nearly died from Ebola, but he managed to live, and the antibodies in his blood have allowed thousands to survive and recover. And isn't that a great metaphor for what Jesus did for us? Jesus died, but He overcame it. Now, the antibodies in His blood allow us to do the same. What do we have to fear when His eternal blood covers us?

The final story I will share in this book is a story of

what is yet to come. It is the inheritance we long for: As the famous song goes, "I can only imagine" what it will be like to see Jesus's return, but this promise drives me forward with anticipation. The Bible says that God is able to do far more than we can ask or imagine (Eph. 3:20), and I know that my story is incomplete—the real thing will always be better. But imagining what it will be like when Jesus comes back helps me run into the fire, not away from it, with unshakeable faith. Please read the scripture and story first, then close your eyes to imagine.

Discussion Questions:

For Individuals or Groups

- How do you feel about running into the fire? What does that mean for you?

- Do you need courage to run into "the fire" today? Pray and ask God to strengthen your faith and help you endure the trials you are going through today.

Six

HEAVEN

"Therefore let us be grateful for receiving a kingdom that cannot be shaken, and thus let us offer to God acceptable worship, with reverence and awe, for our God is a consuming fire." (Heb. 12:28-29)

The light is startling. It bursts from the sky like a thunderstorm. Warm and white, it looks more like the flash of an atomic bomb, except it doesn't cut through me—it glows through me. Suddenly, every muscle in my body relaxes. My jaw loosens, and my hands open. Pain, suffering, sorrow become only shadows of memory of that distant time before this moment.

Everything happens so fast, but it feels like a stop-motion film as I process each change: My hearing is next. I can hear a soft rumbling, like a fresh wind blowing through trees, or a brook bubbling out of everything; prayer is erupting from all around me in every language like a soft roar. It sounds as though the entire Earth is exhaling with a gasp of praise: YHWH.

I become aware of friends and family amidst a huge crowd that goes on for miles, singing and shouting with all their might. Some are holding hands, and some are waving their hands in the air with bursting joy. I see some of the beloved people I've prayed for and witnessed to over my lifetime. Their faces are glowing with joy and love for God. Potent joy, total relief, permeates the air, and I kneel down. I am completely safe. There is no need to watch anymore.

My face is wet. I must have been crying. But I look up, and in an instant I see Him: His hair is white like frosty crystals of snow. His eyes are flames of fire that see everything inside me and still love me. I know those eyes. His feet are like strong, shiny metal, and His voice is like the roar of ocean waves. His face glows like the sun at noon. There are miraculous creatures singing and flying all around Him. I hear my own voice joining with the others, first whispering, then shouting, then singing with all my breath: He is here. King Jesus is here! "Worthy is the Lamb who was slain, to receive power and wealth and wisdom and might and honor and glory and blessing!" (Rev. 5:12). AMEN!

The End

If you would like to be notified when similar books become available, join our reader list at **PorterCreatives.com**.

If you found this book enjoyable, I'd really appreciate it if you wrote a short review since reviews help readers find new books to read. Your help in spreading the word is gratefully appreciated.

Thank you, and happy reading.

Acknowledgements

I thank God for teaching me through the writing of this book and for helping me understand why these stories were important. Thank you, Lord, for a second chance at life.

I am grateful to my husband, who listened to my stories and pitfalls. Thank you for putting God first in our lives and for not being afraid to do what God calls us to do; I love you dearly and thank God for bringing us together. Special thanks to my children for their faith and love for God, and for always telling me that I'm their #1 Mom no matter what.

To my parents, thank you for praying and urging me to tell my story. Thanks to all of my family for patiently cheering me on. Special thanks to the one who threatened to kill me if I dropped out of nursing school.

I especially want to thank my church family—past and present—for praying for me all these years. Special thanks to my mentor for teaching me when I was young and green, and for being willing to talk about spiritual things on the clinical unit.

To all my colleagues: It was an honor to work with you, and I am humbled by the sacrifices you make for others. You practice the greatest commandment to love others more than yourselves, and I am grateful for your example.

Finally, thank you to my readers, who give purpose and perspective to my writing: May God bless you with wisdom and grant you peace.